GROW YOUR OWN DRUGS

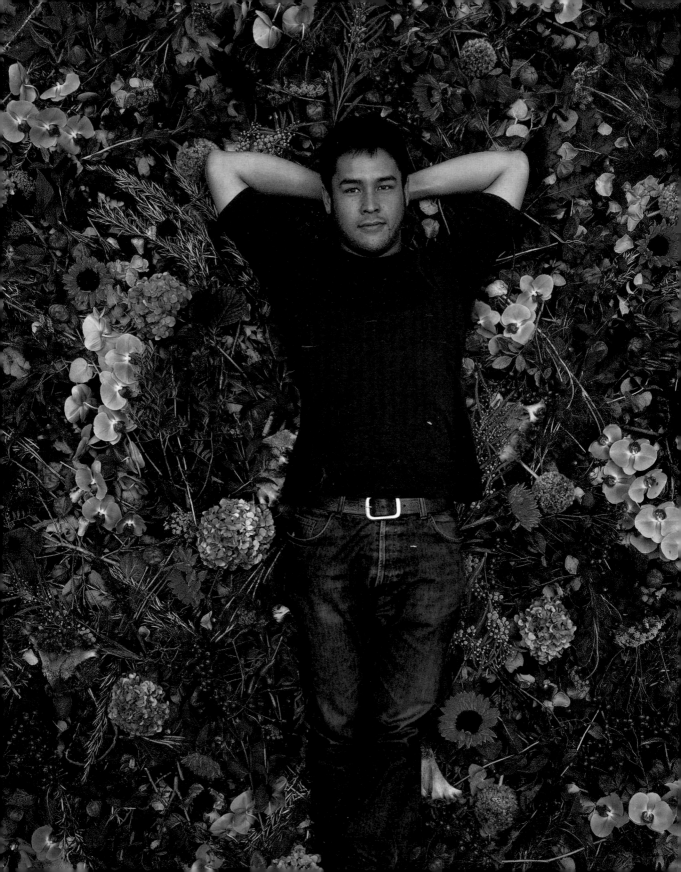

GROW YOUR OWN
DRUGS

Easy recipes for natural remedies and beauty fixes

JAMES WONG

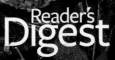

Reader's Digest

The Reader's Digest Association, Inc.
Pleasantville, New York/Montreal/Sydney/Mumbai

A READER'S DIGEST BOOK

First published in 2009 by Collins, an imprint of HarperCollins Publishers
77–85 Fulham Palace Road
Hammersmith
London W6 8JB
www.collins.co.uk

FOR COLLINS

Text by Jane Phillimore
Commissioned photography: Noel Murphy
Design and art direction: Smith & Gilmour
Editor: Caroline Curtis
Food Stylist: Annie Rigg
Stylists: Jo Harris, Nel Haynes

Consultant: Liz Williamson, Professor of Pharmacy, University of Reading
Horticultural Adviser: Michael Kerr
Additional recipes by Richard Adams, Hananja Brice-Ytsma, and Nathalie Chidley of the Archway Clinic of Herbal Medicine,
and by Liz Williamson
Recipe Testing: Nathalie Chidley

FOR READER'S DIGEST
Canadian Project Editor: Pamela Chichinskas
Project Production Coordinator: Wayne Morrison
Senior Art Director: George McKeon
Executive Editor, Trade Publishing: Dolores York
Associate Publisher, Trade Publishing: Rosanne McManus
President and Publisher, Trade Publishing: Harold Clarke

Wong, James.
    Grow your own drugs : easy recipes for natural remedies and beauty fixes / James Wong.
        p. cm.
    Originally published: London : Collins, 2009.
    Includes index.
    ISBN 978-1-60652-107-6
1. Medicinal plants. 2. Materia medica, Vegetable. 3. Toilet preparations. I. Title.
QK99.W66 2009
615'.321--dc22
                            2009030711

We are committed to both the quality of our products and the service we provide to our customers. We value your comments,
so please feel free to contact us.

    The Reader's Digest Association, Inc.
    Adult Trade Publishing
    Reader's Digest Road
    Pleasantville, NY 10570-7000

NOTE TO OUR READERS
The information in this book should not be substituted for, or used to alter, medical therapy without your doctor's advice. For a
specific health problem, consult your physician for guidance. Before using any of these remedies, especially if you have an existing
medical condition, are taking medication, or are pregnant or breast-feeding, check with your physician. Some herbs may interact
with prescription drugs, including the Pill and antidepressants; always do a 24-hour skin test before using. The publishers and
author cannot accept responsibility for any damage incurred as a result of any of the therapeutic methods contained in this work.

For more Reader's Digest products and information, visit our website:
    www.rd.com (in the United States)
    www.readersdigest.ca (in Canada)
    www.readersdigest.com.au (in Australia)
    www.readersdigest.com.nz (in New Zealand)
    www.rdasia.com (in Asia)

Printed in Great Britain by Butler Tanner and Dennis Ltd, Frome and London

3 5 7 9 10 8 6 4 2

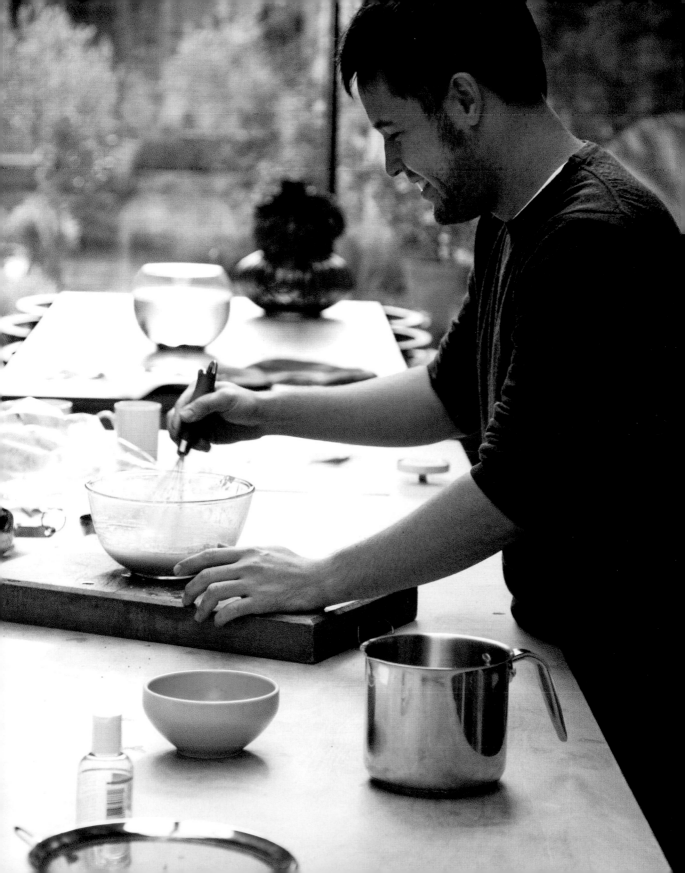

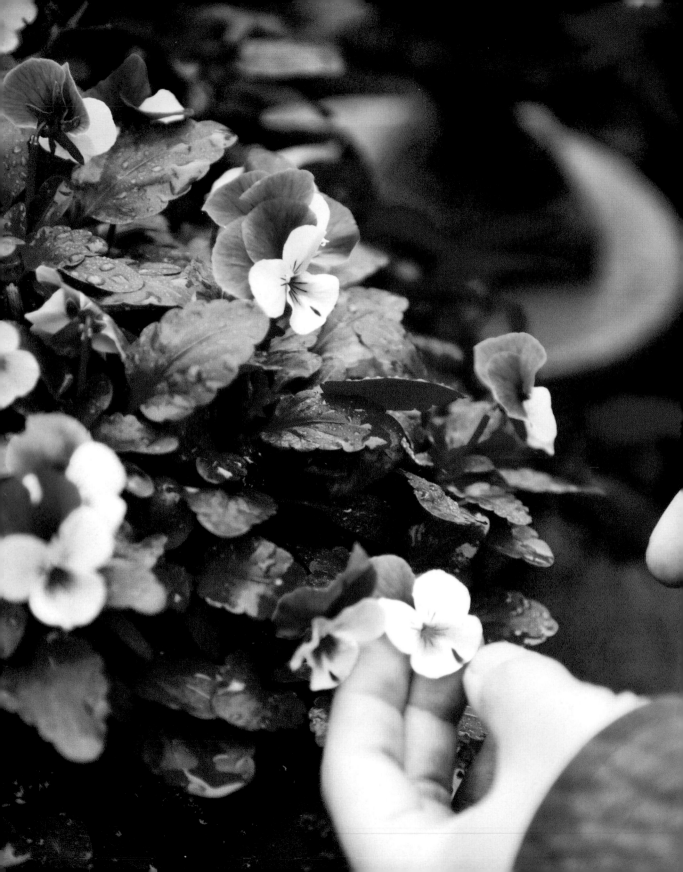

CONTENTS

PREFACE

To the uninitiated, plants probably seem like frivolous decoration, something to brighten up a windowsill or add a splash of color to outdoor spaces. For thousands of kids, being dragged around endless shelves of bedding plants each spring has all the appeal of shopping for curtains. So it's not surprising that my friends think my plant obsession is possibly the least cool of all interests—and looking at it from their perspective, I must say I agree with them.

What none of them realizes, however, is that this perception of plants as purely ornamental objects is a strange cultural anomaly that has existed in only one civilization in history—our own. In every other culture, the plants that surround us are a living supermarket, pharmacy, a home improvement center, and even a liquor store—all rolled into one. In just a couple of generations, we in the West have become vastly unacquainted with the varied and vitally important uses of the botanical world. The irony, however, is that we are just as reliant on plants for all aspects of our daily survival as we have ever been—we just don't seem to know it. Plants are not only responsible for the air we breathe but also for the food we eat and the stability of the planet's very climate. They are the basis of a large part of our medicine, with up to 50 percent of the world's top proprietary drugs originally derived from natural sources.

As an ethnobotanist, I am trained to look beyond the aesthetic and to see plants for what they really are—the chemical factories that make all life on Earth possible. When I walk around a garden center, I see a kind of living pharmacy collected together from all over the world—the leaves of an assassin's poison on one shelf, the flowers of a ritual hallucinogen on another, or a cutting-edge antimalarial growing as a weed in the pot of a common garden tree that is currently being analyzed for use in the treatment of cancer. When looked at this way, plants become warehouses of infinite possibility. Understanding the medicinal uses of the plants around us does not require some superhuman (or should that be supergeeky?) ability but is actually the way in which every other culture on Earth sees plants—the way, in fact, that all of us did until a few short decades ago. Many of these beliefs aren't just old wives' tales or a last bit of mumbo jumbo that has yet to be swept away by reason and science. Traditional plant-based remedies have provided modern Western medicine with some of its most important drugs, and they are still being studied by pharmaceutical companies for properties that may lead to new breakthroughs. Indeed, the natural origins behind major drugs such as aspirin, morphine, penicillin, and even contraceptive pills reveal that "natural" medicine is not as separate from "conventional" medicine as it is popularly conceived to be. In fact, the World Health Organization estimates that up to 80 percent of the world's population relies on plant-based medicine as the key form of health care and actively promotes its use.

In many ways, I feel fortunate that I first experienced plants not as simply decorative but as an intrinsic part of my everyday life in rural Malaysia. I remember sitting, fascinated, on the kitchen floor with my grandmother, watching as she poured mixtures of pungent spices and brightly colored roots from her garden into a huge stone mortar and pestle. She then ground them into a fragrant mush to make tonics—though I also found, much to her horror, that her mush made a great face paint. Her plants and remedies were always on hand, whether it was small bottles of camphor (*Cinnamomum camphora*) and eucalyptus (*Eucalyptus globulus*) oil whipped out of her handbag to take the itch out of mosquito bites at the Chinese New Year's fireworks display or the bright red orchid (*Bletilla chinensis*) roots lifted from her backyard and boiled to make a spicy chicken soup when I had a cold.

I was brought up to see plants as solutions in life rather than as just a pretty backdrop to it—and I hope this book provides a glimpse into this traditional way of looking at plants.

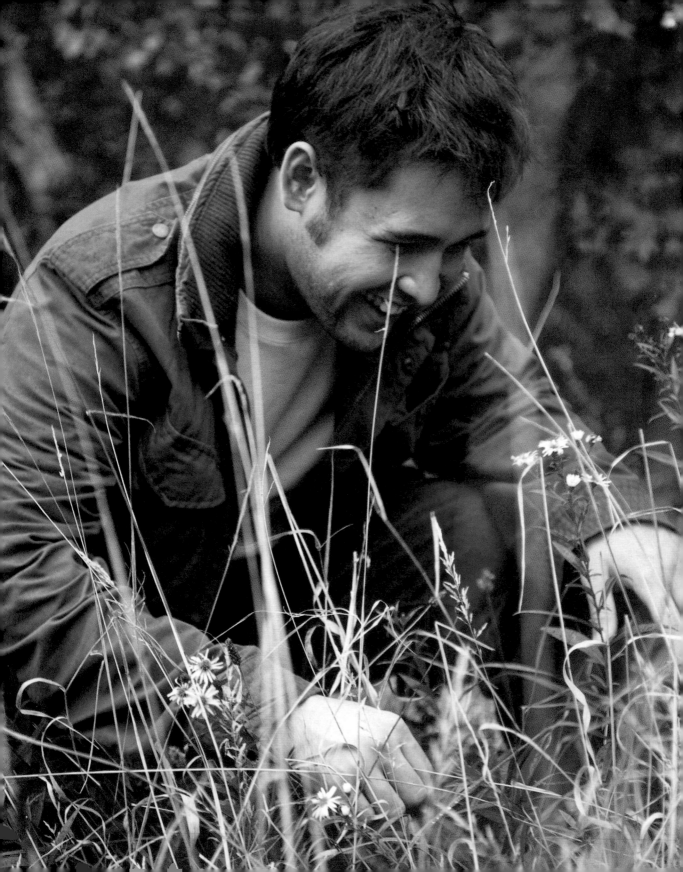

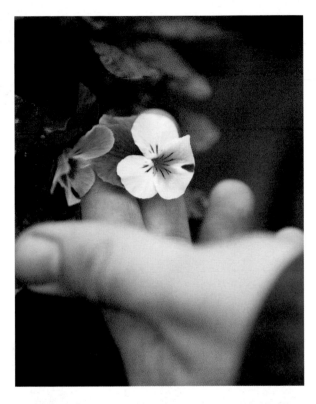

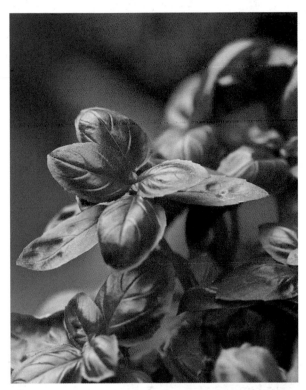

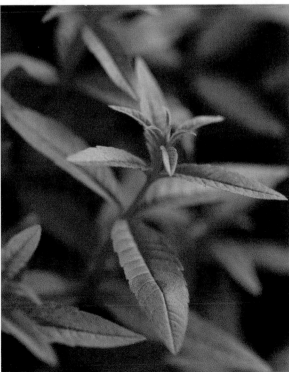

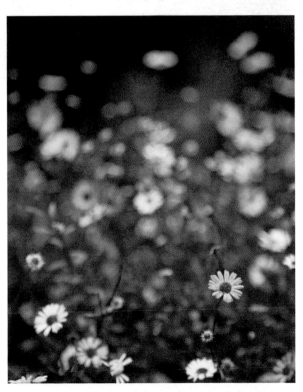

INTRODUCTION

In the last few years, there's been a surge of interest in using herbs and plants to treat common ailments. Many people consider plant-based remedies to be more natural, cheaper, and less harmful to the body than pharmaceutical drugs and more capable of easing both everyday and chronic health problems, which conventional medicine often finds difficult to treat.

At least, that's the theory; the reality is not quite so straightforward. Yes, there's a long history of using plants to treat disease, but until the twentieth century, these were the only medicines available, and the herbal remedies that have been passed down through the generations cannot necessarily be relied upon. Across the globe there are up to 50,000 plants used medicinally, and we're constantly being bombarded with "wonder" claims for the latest, often pricey, herbal cures. So how can you tell which plants work and which don't? And which you can grow at home?

This book provides some of the answers. First and foremost, *Grow Your Own Drugs* is a guide to help you get the most out of plants and their various properties. It explains how to grow and harvest suitable plants in your backyard and then make them into simple, effective remedies to treat a range of common ailments. There are over sixty recipes for teas, tinctures, creams, lotions, balms, gargles, and cough syrups—all easy, inexpensive, and fun to make. And just in case your vanity is looking bare, there are also lots of natural alternatives to your existing beauty products, from moisturizers and lip balms to bath bombs and face packs.

In the second half of this book, the section Top 100 medicinal Plants offers first-class horticultural information as well as scientific insights into the plants, flowers, fruits, and roots you'll encounter on your herbal journey. How plants can improve health is currently the subject of much scientific analysis. This book distills the knowledge of herbal practitioners with the most up-to-date scientific findings to bring you practical and reliable information about these plants and the natural remedies made from them. The majority of these plants will happily root in your backyard, but I have also included a few exotic, tender specimens because they are such outstanding performers. You may not be able to grow these yourself, but you will be able to find the essential oils or extracts, as well as dried herbs, on sale in natural food stores or online.

Safety is a primary concern when using plant material. Although some of these treatments may give over-the-counter medicines a run for their money, it is important that you don't diagnose or medicate yourself or others without first seeking medical advice. This is particularly true if you have an existing medical condition, are taking medication, or are pregnant. Check with your family doctor before using these remedies. If you think you may be sensitive to any of the ingredients, try a 24-hour skin test first, because some people can have adverse reactions. Equally important is the need to make sure you have identified the species correctly: Certain plants, even those closely related to medicinal species, can be poisonous or deadly.

Using plant-based remedies is a fascinating way to look after your family's health. It's a great pleasure to be in touch with nature, to grow and harvest your own plants, and to make your own remedies. Nowadays, we're lucky enough to have the best of both medical worlds. Modern medicine is hugely effective in the treatment of serious diseases, but plant-based remedies give us gentle ways to manage everyday ailments and keep ourselves in optimum health. After reading this book, you'll never look at your backyard the same way again.

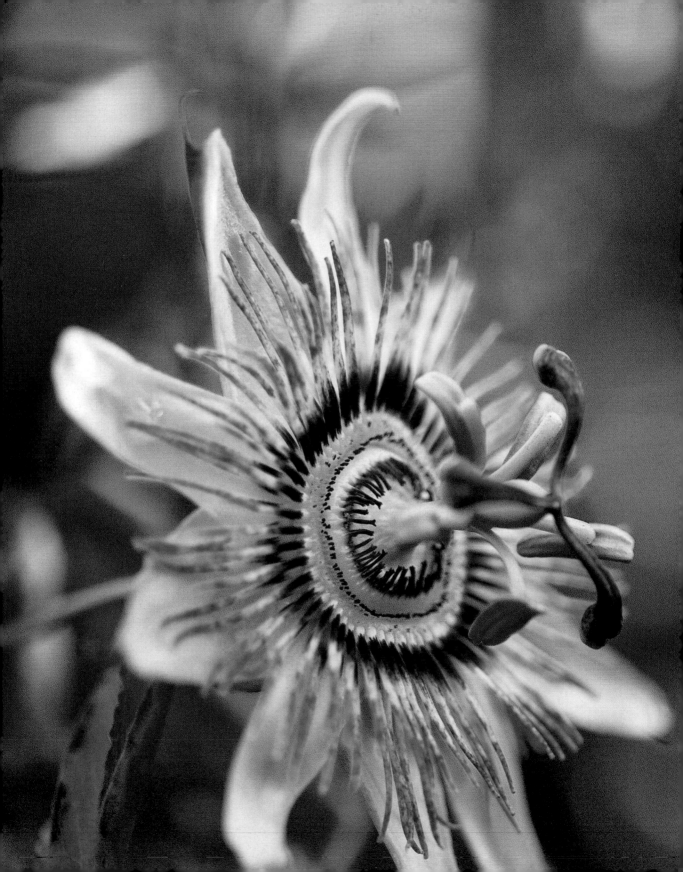

getting started

After reading the labels of the natural remedies and organic cosmetic products found in natural food stores, you may think you need to scour the Amazon for rare plants or own a state-of-the-art laboratory to prepare herbal remedies. The reality is, however, natural remedies are almost always made from the most common backyard plants, prepared on top of the kitchen stove in a matter of minutes.

It is important to remember that traditional plant-based medicine is a system of health care that evolved in societies where people did not always have a great deal of money, time, or resources. The indigenous women I studied in rural Ecuador as part of the research for my master's degree, for example, couldn't go trekking into the mountains for herbs and then spend hours grinding, boiling, filtering, and drying these each time one of their children had a headache. With up to eight other children to take care of, they needed to find effective solutions within their immediate environment. Solutions that were inexpensive, easy, and quick to prepare—basically made from the contents of their backyard. The parallels with our own time-starved way of life in Western society are obvious.

All you need to get started are the basic tools of any kitchen, as well as access to plant material, whether that's in a tiny window box, your local supermarket, or from the weeds growing in your lawn. Quite literally, if your kitchen facilities and cooking ability can stretch to making grilled cheese, you will be able to make herbal remedies. Now go on and get started!

YOUR PANTRY

Making herbal remedies is just like cooking, and you'll probably find you already have most of the basic ingredients on your kitchen shelves. Staples like olive oil, sea salt, honey, cider or wine vinegar, and baking soda are the basis for many of these recipes. However, there are also a few extra ingredients you'll need to keep on hand, especially if you want to make creams, balms, and lotions.

Beeswax and Emulsifying Wax

Lotions and creams are essentially made up of oil and water, but as every schoolchild knows, oil and water don't mix. Something extra—a wax or other emulsifier—is needed to "glue" and bind the cream together. Emulsifiers work at a molecular level by attracting and trapping water and oil. They also thicken the mix to create a lotion or cream that can be smoothed into skin.

Beeswax, whether white or yellow, is a natural emulsifier taken from honeycombs, the internal walls of a hive. It is antibacterial, as well as being an excellent skin softener, soother, and moisture retainer. You can buy it online as granules, pellets, or solid wax. (You can also use beeswax candles or beeswax furniture polish as long as these are labeled 100 percent pure beeswax.)

Emulsifying waxes are synthetically produced and used in most over-the-counter cosmetic products. There are many different kinds, most of which are suitable for vegans. They usually come as granules, which melt quickly and can be bought online.

Essential Oils

Some recipes use essential plant oils. These add fragrance, and many also have medicinal properties—for example, tea tree oil is an antibacterial. However, they are extremely concentrated and, as a rule, should never be taken internally. If undiluted oils get on your skin, be sure to wash off immediately.

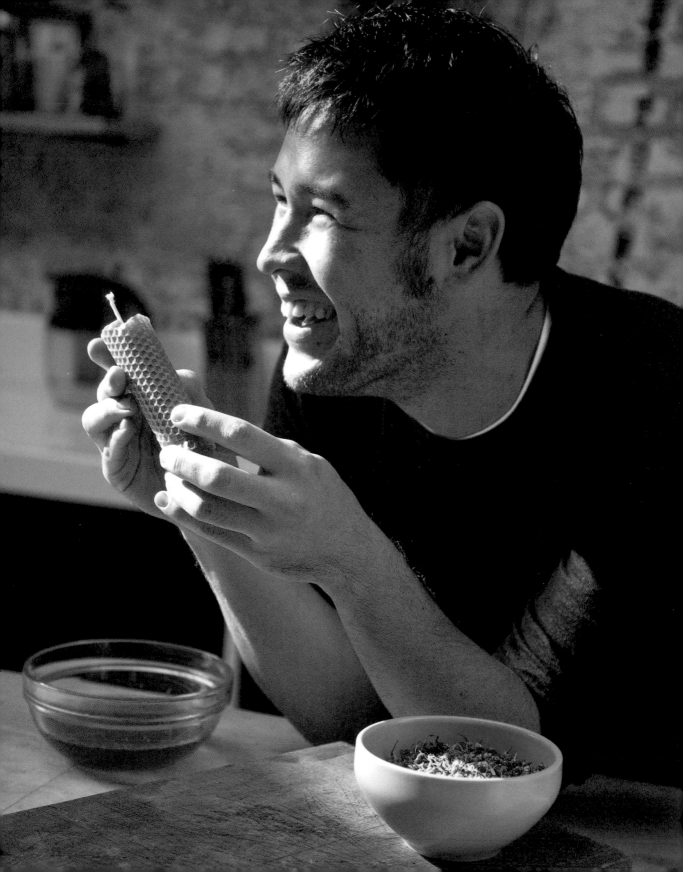

Gelatin

Gelatin is a clear thickening and setting agent used to make gels. Powdered gelatin is easiest to use, dissolved in cold or slightly warm water—boiling water impairs its setting qualities. You can also buy animal-based or vegetable gelatin from supermarkets.

Glycerin

Glycerin is a clear, odorless liquid that can be used to make tinctures for children or adults who don't want alcohol-based ones. (Bear in mind, though, that these tinctures have a shorter shelf life than alcohol-based tinctures.) Glycerin is slightly sweet and has soothing properties, so it is often used in over-the-counter products for sore throats and intestinal disorders. It is also used in the preparation of creams, lotions, and syrups as a thickener and preserving agent.

Oils

The base oil for these recipes is usually olive oil, sunflower oil, or almond oil (which is good for topical use because it is high in vitamin E). Other oils—such as wheatgerm, avocado, sesame, and coconut—have specific properties that are useful in certain remedies. Always choose a fresh, good-quality oil that has been stored in a cool, dark place—oils can go rancid quickly.

Vitamin C Powder

Vitamin C is a powerful antioxidant that acts as a natural preservative. It is commonly used in skin creams.

Suppliers

Most of these products are available in supermarkets and health food stores (see Resources, page 218).

CREATE AN OUTDOOR PHARMACY

Where do you find the plants to harvest and make plant-based remedies? You can grow most in your garden at home; others you will be able to forage from meadows, roadsides, or in the wild. Many plants used in these recipes grow so freely that they are classified as weeds—chickweed, dandelion, nettles, and plantain spring to mind.

Fresh versus Dried

Most of the recipes in this book use fresh plant material wherever possible, so you can grow, pick, and use your own directly from the garden, ensuring that all the active ingredients are present in the maximum amounts. However, because fresh plant material is unobtainable at certain times of the year, you may have to use dried herbs instead. If herbs have been dried carefully and thoroughly, they can be used just as effectively as fresh. Drying your own is easy—see How to Dry Plants, page 37. Some dried plants are a little different from fresh—think of the change in ginger when it is dried—but this is fairly unusual.

When using dried herbs in a recipe, use only about half the amount specified for fresh plant material, because the dried is more concentrated.

Growing at Home

Even if you don't have your own garden, you can use pots and window boxes for growing a surprisingly large number of these plants, even small shrubs and trees. For example, a fig tree grows well in a good-sized pot; in fact, restricting its roots in this way makes it produce bigger fruit and more of it. Plants that do well in pots include:

> Most small herbs, including caraway, dill, lemon balm, all the mints, parsley, and sage.
> Fruits and vegetables such as cranberries, goji berries, chili peppers, garlic, watercress, and wheatgrass.
> Flowers like lavender, marigold (*Calendula officinalis*), nasturtium, and rose geranium.
> Roots like ginger and horseradish.

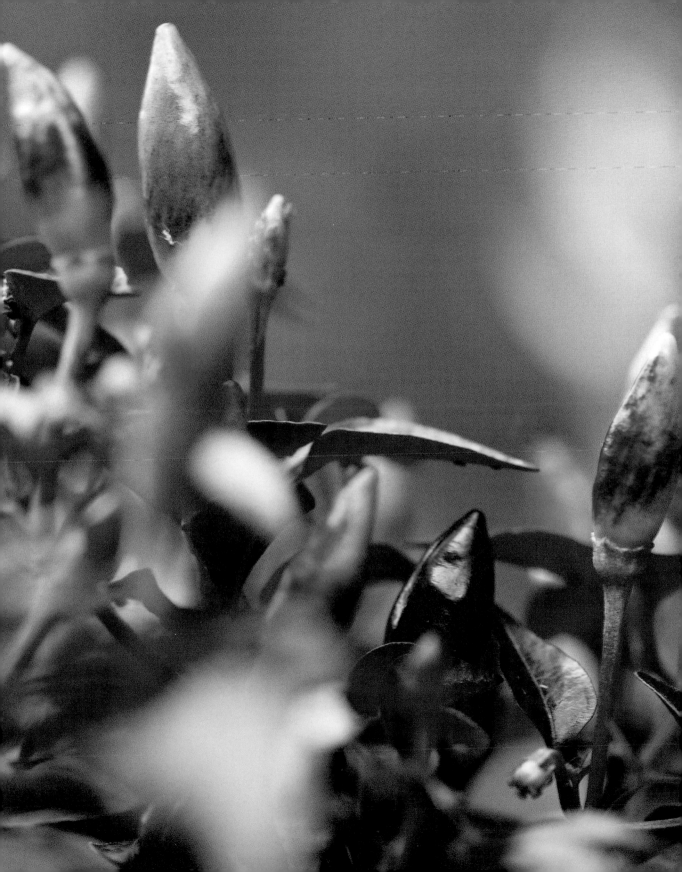

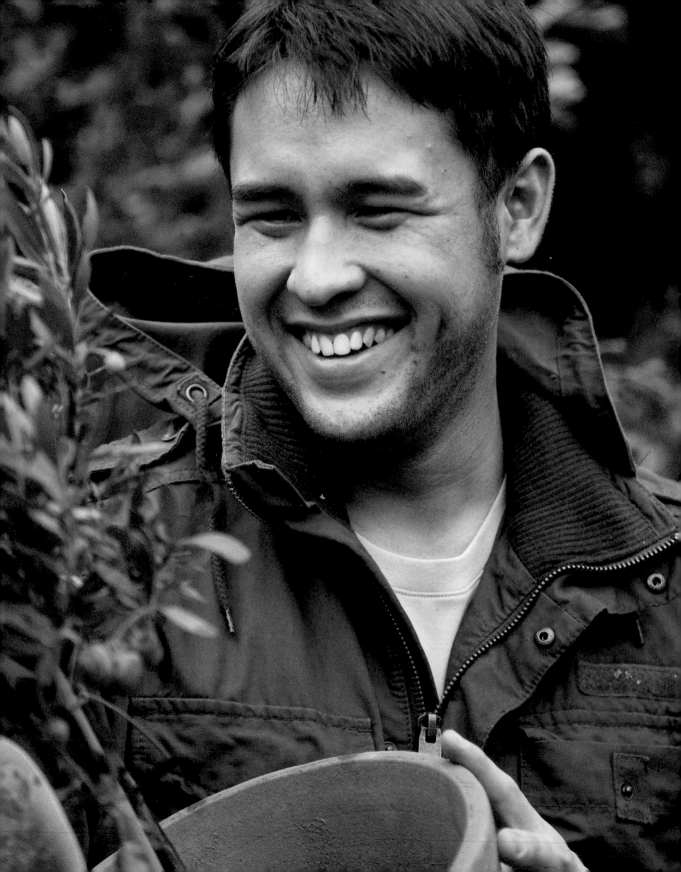

> Small trees like fig or cultivars of spruce and cypress ('Amber Glow,' 'Caespitosa,' or 'Tiny Tim'), as long as the pots are large.

The biggest danger with pots is drought: The soil dries out quickly, especially in highly porous terra-cotta pots, leaving the roots searching around to find water in a very confined space. Water and feed the soil in pots regularly during the growing season from spring to summer, but be careful to keep the potting mix from drying out in winter (overwatering is as big a killer as underwatering in indoor plants). Weather permitting, put pots outside on balconies, porches, or window ledges to catch the sun, and choose frost-resistant containers that won't crack and expose roots to freezing temperatures.

HERB GARDEN TOP 10

Even in the smallest garden, you can create a complete medicinal herb patch. With space at a premium, you need to make sure that each plant is really earning its keep.

These are the 10 plants that are as versatile as they are effective:

Chamomille (*Matricaria recutita*)—soothes indigestion and colic, eases tension, and is good for skin irritations.

Echinacea—boosts the immune system and lessens the severity of colds and flu.

Johnny-jump-up (*Viola tricolor*)—has anti-inflammatory properties; good for eczema and skin blemishes; loosens phlegm.

Lavender—calms and relaxes, eases pain, and when applied to cuts and bruises functions as an antiseptic.

Lemon balm—soothes nervous tension and anxiety, promotes sleep, and speeds the healing of cold sores.

Marigold (*Calendula officinalis*)—good for sunburn, acne, and blemishes; soothes ulcers and digestive problems.

Peppermint—good for digestion, gas, and headaches.

Rosemary—helps memory and concentration, improves mood, and sweetens breath.

Sage—good for coughs, colds and congestion, and hot flushes.

St.-John's-wort—works as an antidepressant and promotes skin healing.

If you have a greenhouse, you can boost the contents of your herbal cabinet by growing useful but tender plants such as ginger and cucumber. If a windowsill is your only option, an aloe vera plant is ideal.

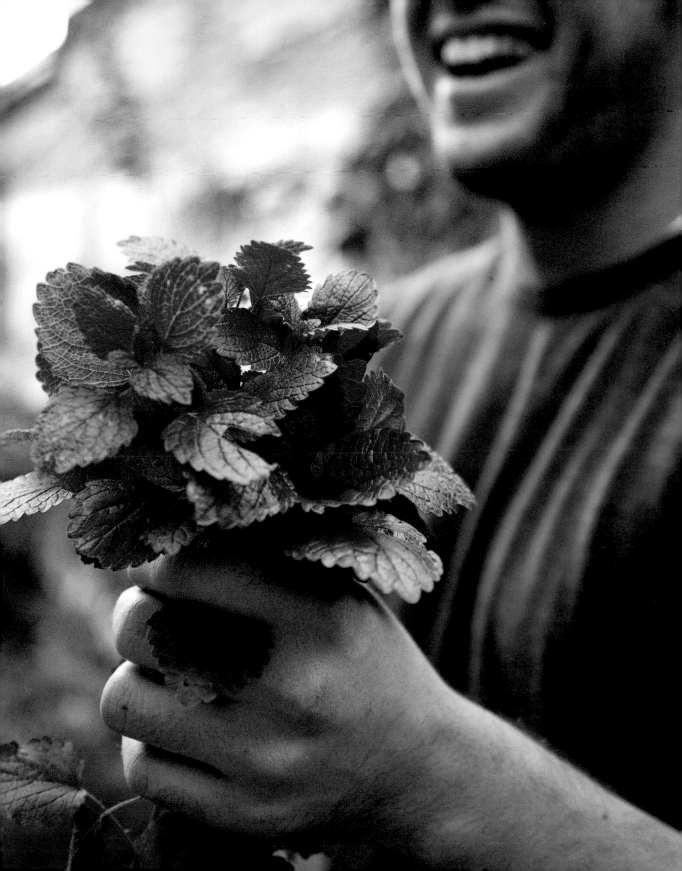

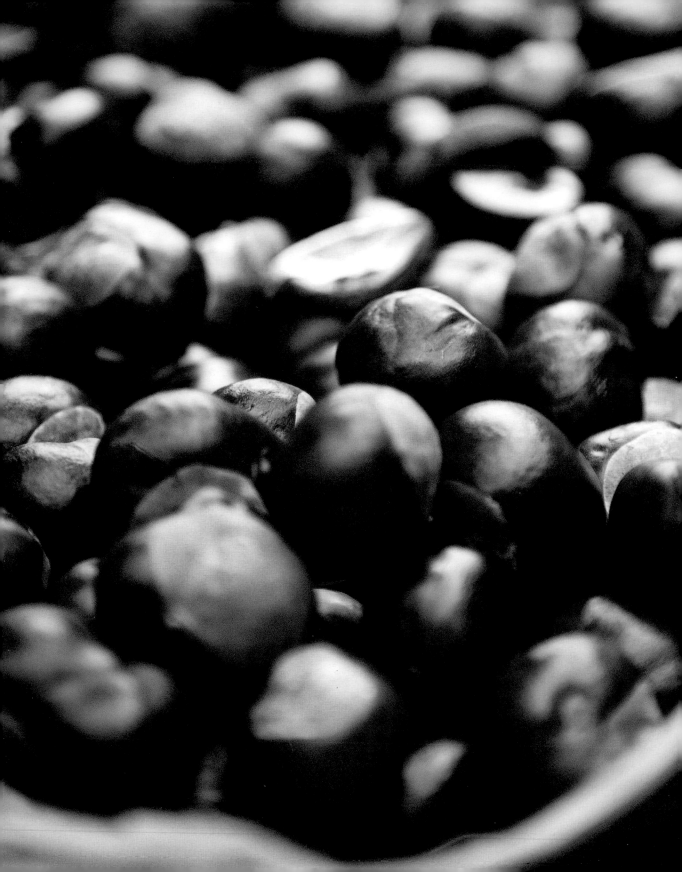

Buying Plants

Most plants can be grown from seed or purchased at your local garden center. Less common plants and trees can be sourced from specialized nurseries or online.

In the Wild

Many of the plants in this book are plentiful and can be found growing in the fields or even on empty lots in towns and cities. For example, the seeds of horse chestnuts may be found in your local park in September and October and yarrow in meadows during summer months.

Best Time for Harvesting

Leaves—gather leaves throughout the growing season (usually spring to fall). If you want to harvest large amounts of a certain plant, cut back in early summer to half its height, leaving enough regrowth time for a second cutting later in the year.

Flowers—pick as soon as possible after they open.

Roots—harvest in the fall, when the roots have stored the most food and essential compounds.

Fruits and Seeds—pick when they ripen to a mature color, but before they shrivel or decay.

Plants grow in a variety of habitats in North America and can sometimes be found in surprising places. It's worth keeping your eyes open for foraging opportunities wherever you are.

Foraging Rules

Be sure to check with local authorities before you gather fruit, flowers, and foliage in the wild for personal use. Below are a few guidelines that should always be followed when harvesting plants:

> Don't pick anything unless you're absolutely sure of its identity. It is very easy to confuse two plants that look alike or have similar names; for example, harmless, edible, sweet cicely (*Myrrhis odorata*) and toxic hemlock (*Conium maculatum*) look very similar. Take a well-illustrated field guide with you to help identify plants.

> Don't pick alongside busy roads or on agricultural land, because the plants are likely to be polluted or sprayed with pesticides and chemical fertilizers. Remember, pesticides can travel a large distance in the wind so it is important to find out about chemical use in your area before doing any picking.

> Don't pick plants that look diseased or stunted; select the healthiest specimens you can find.

> Harvest only as much as you will use, and don't take more than half the leaves, fruit, or stems of any plant. Always leave enough for wildlife to eat and to ensure future plant generations. If there's not enough of a plant to leave some of it behind, then don't pick it.

> Check with the local property owner before digging anything up: You have a legal obligation to get permission first. Also, it is illegal to remove plants from a national park.

> Don't dig up roots unless they are from a prolific plant, such as dandelion. Also be sure not to harvest too many roots from any one area.

> Never pick a rare or endangered species. You can download a rare-plant register from the website of the U.S. Department of Agriculture (http://plants.usa.gov/) or the Committee on the Status of Endangered Wildlife in Canada (www.cosewic.gc.ca).

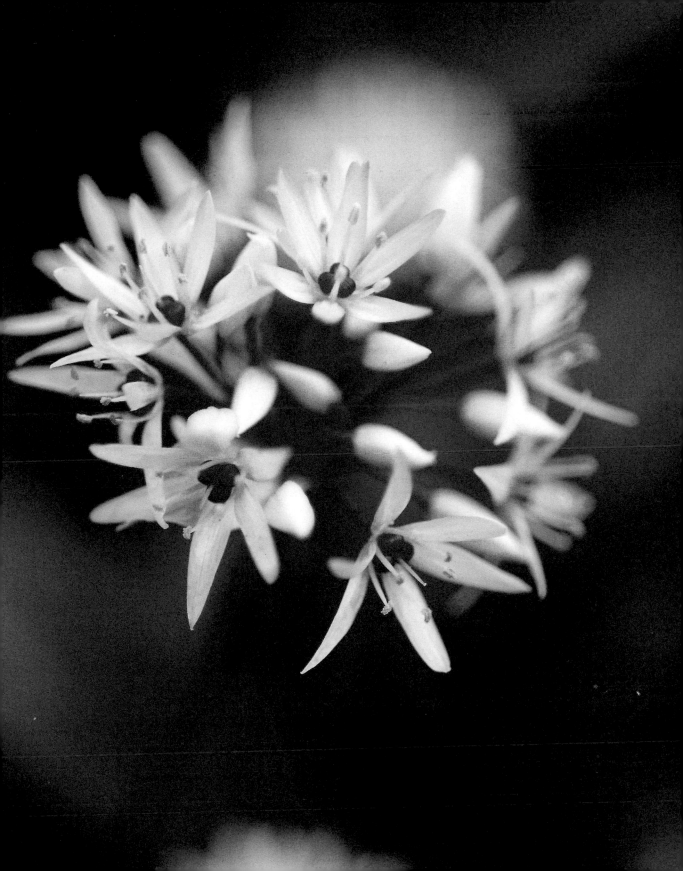

Foraging Supplies

For the basics to get you started, you will need a canvas bag or backpack and a pair of scissors. Foraging enthusiasts may want to add the following items to their bag:

> pruning shears
> trowel or small hand shovel (for roots)
> knife
> carrier bags or garden trugs to carry stems, flowers, and leaves
> paper bags to keep seeds dry and cool
> sealed plastic containers to keep fruit from getting bruised
> gardening gloves

Remember to keep your arms and legs covered to protect yourself from poison ivy, insect bites, and thorns.

USEFUL EQUIPMENT

You won't need any special equipment for making these remedies, although a few basic kitchen utensils will come in handy:

> teapot with a lid to make tisanes and infusions
> kitchen scale
> measuring cup
> glass mixing bowls of various sizes
> saucepans of various sizes
> fine-meshed sieve and colander
> blender
> wire whisk
> wooden spoon and large metal spoon

You may also find it helpful to keep the following items on hand:

Mortar and Pestle—Leaves, roots, and seeds should be as fresh as possible, so it's always best to grind your own. You can use a mortar and pestle or a manual coffee grinder or pepper mill. If you opt for the coffee grinder or pepper mill, dedicate it solely for this use or you will end up with an awful-tasting mixture of ground herbs and coffee/pepper.

Pan and Glass Bowl—Plants, oils, and wax must be heated slowly and evenly; the best way to do this is in a double boiler, or bain-marie (a pan in which water is heated, with a bowl placed on top to hold the ingredients). Beeswax can leave a nasty residue, so if you're making regular batches of creams, you may want to invest in a dedicated pan and bowl set.

Cheesecloth—You will find this invaluable for straining herbs. Fold cheesecloth in two and line in a sieve or colander. Then strain infusions and oils through it. Squeeze out excess juice by twisting the cloth in your hands.

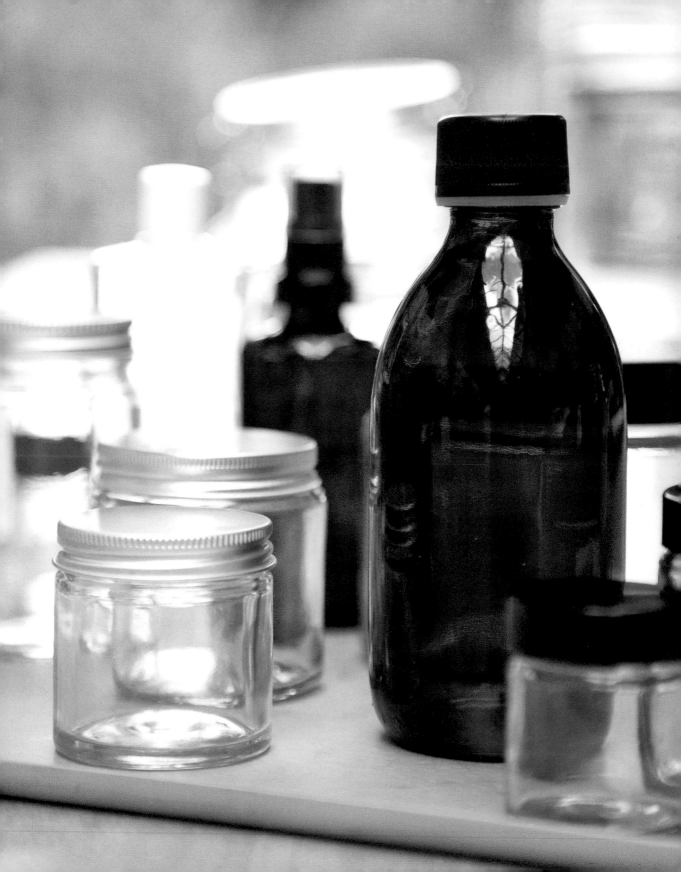

Glass Jars—Gather an assortment of all shapes and sizes, new or recycled. Canning jars with tight-fitting lids are good for macerating oils; syrup bottles for storing syrups and soothing cough mixtures; and small, wide-mouthed jars for salves and ointments. You can get screw, stopper, and spray tops, or pipette and dropper tops for tiny dosages. Glass usually comes clear or colored (amber, blue, brown, black). Clear glass is good for storing herbs (you can easily check for fading and color changes, which are signs of deterioration). Dark glass is better for storing oils and tinctures over long periods of time, because it offers protection from light.

Before you bottle a preparation, always sterilize jars by washing them, along with the lids, in very hot water. Then rinse well. Place on a cookie sheet lined with paper. Turn your oven to 150°F (70°C) and place the cookie sheet inside for at least 20 minutes. This will dry and warm the jars before filling. Alternatively, you can put the jars through the hottest dishwasher cycle.

Filters and Funnels—Getting hot liquid into bottles is easier using these. Metal or plastic filters and funnels work well and are available in a variety of sizes at kitchen stores.

Adhesive Labels—Labels come in a variety of sizes and shapes, plain or with with colorful designs. Once you have filled the jar, prepare a label by recording the name of what's inside, the date, dosage, and storage details. It's important that you dispose of the treatments after the recommended storage time.

Notebook—Record your experiences: where and when you picked the plants, your favorite recipes, what you liked/didn't like about them, suppliers' details, etc.

USING PLANTS

You can use plant-based remedies internally as teas, oils, vinegars, and syrups, or apply them externally as creams, balms, bath/massage oils, and poultices.

Tea or Infusion—like making a cup of tea

The simplest way to extract the essential constituents of fresh leaves and flowers is by making an infusion. Place the washed, chopped plants in a glass bowl, pour freshly boiled water over (about 30 g of fresh plants to 2 cups (500 ml) of water; or 15 g of dried plant material). Let stand, covered, for 8 to 10 minutes, or until the water takes on color. Strain through a sieve lined with cheesecloth. Drink the same day, pour into a bath, or use in lotions and creams.

Decoction—like making tea but leaving it to simmer

The roots, bark, and woody parts of a plant need to be left to simmer to extract the essential ingredients, a process called decoction. Wash and chop the root, place in a pan, and add water (about 30 g of fresh root to 2 cups (500 ml) of water). Cover the pan and bring to a boil, then simmer for at least 10 minutes. Strain through a sieve lined with cheesecloth. Drink the same day, pour into a bath, or use in lotions and creams.

Tinctures—chopped plants steeped in alcohol

A tincture uses alcohol to extract the essential compounds from plants. This method is highly effective, especially for fibrous plants, roots, and resins. Vodka is the alcohol of choice, being colorless and almost flavorless; however, rum, brandy, and whisky may also be used. Make sure the alcohol is 80 proof (that is, 40 percent alcohol) or the tincture may turn moldy in the bottle.

To make a tincture, fill a jar with plant material and cover with alcohol. Run a knife down the sides of the jar to dispel any air bubbles. Seal and leave in a dark, cool place for 8 days to 1 month, shaking occasionally. When ready, strain through a cheesecloth-lined sieve and pour into small bottles. Alcohol is a preservative, so tinctures have a longer shelf life than other preparations, keeping for up to 5 years.

Infused Oils—like making tea but using oil instead of water

Infused or macerated oils—in which plants are left in a base oil for up to 2 weeks to extract their essential compounds—are used to make creams, lotions, and massage oils for external or sometimes even internal use. To infuse oil, fill a jar with plant material and cover with oil. Run a knife down the sides of the inside to dispel air bubbles. Seal and leave in a warm place for 2 weeks, or until the oil has taken on color; then strain and bottle. For a quicker maceration, place the herbs and oil in a pan and cook over a low heat for about 20 minutes; then strain and bottle. Infused oils will last from 6 months to 1 year.

Salves and Balms

To make a lip salve, ointment, or balm, add beeswax to an infused oil and heat gently to melt. The waxy mixture will solidify as it cools. Lip salves and balms are thicker than ointments, which are generally applied over a larger area of the body. Check to see whether the mixture is the consistency you want by spooning a few drops into a glass of ice water. A thick salve will form into a little ball; a thinner ointment will disperse over the surface. You can thicken by adding more beeswax (½ tsp at a time) or thin by adding more oil (1 tsp at a time), testing again until you get the desired consistency. When ready, pour while still warm into wide-mouthed jars for easy use. Salves will last 1 to 2 years.

Creams and Lotions

These are emulsions, made by mixing a water-based and oil-based preparation together over heat and "glueing" them together with an emulsifier, like beeswax or emulsifying wax. Creams and lotions made this way feel wonderfully smooth on the skin, but they have a shorter shelf life than salves. They will last in the refrigerator for up to 2 months.

Gels

These are used to make skin preparations such as gels or face masks. Gels are made by dissolving gelatin with an infusion or juice. They should be used right away; if you wish to store for a longer period, add alcohol or essential oils.

Herb-Infused Honey

Honey acts as an antibacterial agent and can be applied topically to wounds. Herb-infused honey is very easy to make: Simply heat the herbs with honey for about 1 hour, then bottle. Honey is often used as a throat soother and to help with congestion in the upper respiratory tract. Naturally sweet, herb honey is an ideal means for encouraging children to take herbs: Spread on toast or give a spoonful every day. Herb-infused honey will last for up to 6 months.

Syrups and Lozenges

Cough syrups are like runny jams, made by boiling a plant in water with sugar or honey, sometimes with gelatin added as a thickener. These syrups keep well in sterilized jars—from 6 months to 1 year if sealed and unopened and, once opened, for 3 months in the refrigerator. By adding more sugar or boiling for a longer period of time, you can produce a solidified mass that can be broken up into small cough drops for use throughout the day.

Vinegars

When heated with herbs for a few hours, vinegar extracts the essential constituents from plants. Herbal vinegars can be used in cooking, salad dressings, or taken by spoon every day. They may also be used externally as a hair rinse or hair tonic, or added to a bath. Cider or wine vinegar is usually used as the base. Herbal vinegars will keep for approximately 6 months.

Poultices and Compresses

The body can absorb essential compounds through the skin, and applying plant material directly as a poultice can relieve backache, muscle pains, strains, and headaches and can also help to clear skin outbreaks. A simple poultice is made of crushed plants, sometimes mixed in a flour paste. Apply to the skin and cover with gauze and a bandage; change every few hours.

A compress applies plant infusions or decoctions directly to the skin. To make, soak a linen or cotton cloth in a hot or cold plant infusion or decoction. Wring out, then apply. Hot compresses need to be changed regularly.

How to Dry Plants

Drying plants allows you to use them out of season. It is important that dried plants not contain too much residual water or they will turn muddy. They should be dried quickly but without too much heat and should be kept out of direct sunlight to avoid destroying the active compounds. To dry plants, select one of the following two methods:

Air-Drying—Gather loose, leafy bunches of plants, then tie with string or rubber band. Hang upside down (so the oils go into the leaves) in a well-ventilated, dry environment out of direct sunlight. Leave for at least 2 weeks, or until crispy. When ready, strip the leaves/flowers off the stems, then crumble, and store in an airtight colored glass jar or container. Dried this way, herbs will keep for up to 1 year.

Oven-Drying—Cover a cookie sheet with parchment paper and then put the plants on it, spacing them well apart. Place in the oven on the lowest setting, leaving the door slightly open, until dry—this may take up to 5 hours. Crumble and store as above.

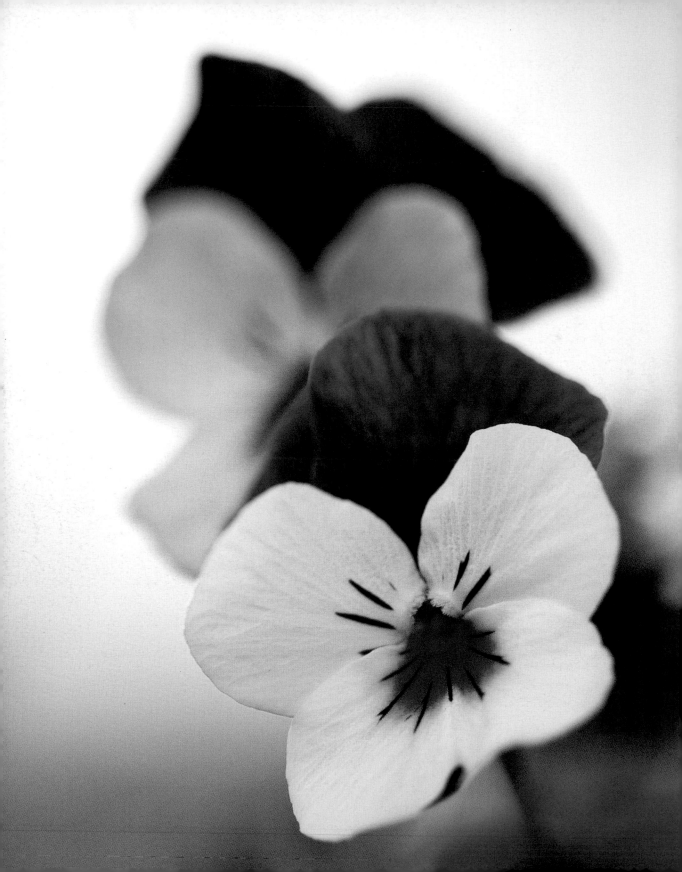

remedies

This is the really fun part. For me, cooking up these concoctions is like returning to my childhood—stirring sticky mixtures, pouring out goopy gels, and playing around with amazing smells, colors, and flavors. The fact that these remedies might be effective in clearing up a breakout of acne, calming anxiety, or even alleviating chronic nausea is just an added bonus.

To make things easy for you, I have broken down these recipes according to the type of complaints each treats and, in many cases, have provided additional recipes for each condition so you can experiment to find out which one works best for you.

Aside from being fun to make, most are straightforward. Indeed, this section is set up like a cookbook. To get started, read through a recipe to check for the ingredients you need and whether it takes a while to macerate (soak). Then you're all set to go. It's a great excuse to get the kids involved, too. What better way to learn about plants and science than to make an explosively fizzy bath bomb?

DIGESTIVE DISORDERS

Bad breath is the scourge of stomach ailments, but thyme is a great healer (excuse the pun). As an essential oil, it contains thymol, a powerful antiseptic used in dentistry. Combined with mint and aniseed, two other big odor busters, it makes an excellent breath freshener.

BAD BREATH
Thyme Sweet Breath Spray and Mouthwash

10 tbsp (approx. 25 g) fresh thyme leaves
10 tbsp (approx. 30 g) fresh mint leaves
5 fresh eucalyptus leaves
3 tsp anise seed
3 tsp cloves
¾ cup (approx. 200 ml) vodka
rind of 1 lemon
1 tbsp sorbitol or other artificial sweetener to taste, if desired
4 tbsp glycerin

1 Strip the thyme, mint, and eucalyptus leaves from their stems and chop. Place in a blender and mix. Add the aniseed and cloves to the blender and mix again.

2 Place in a dark bottle with the vodka, lemon, and sorbitol (if using) and leave for 10 days to 1 month to macerate.

3 Strain through cheesecloth. Add the glycerin, then stir and pour into a small spray bottle (with a yield of up to 1 g per spray).

USE Spray 1 g into the mouth when needed. NOTE: This spray contains alcohol, so be careful not to overuse, especially if driving. Do not use if pregnant.

STORAGE Keeps for up to 1 year.

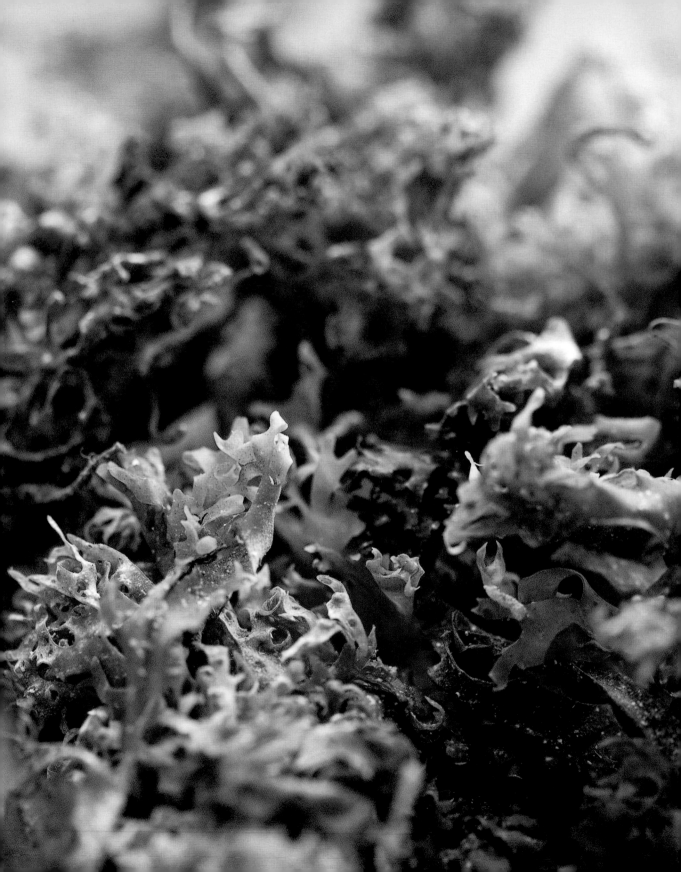

Bloating and belching are common side effects of heartburn and indigestion. At the first sign of any discomfort, take a spoonful of this soothing mixture. The seaweed coats and protects the stomach lining but also floats on top of the stomach contents, acting as a "raft" to calm things down and stop reflux. The mixture also works as an antacid, thanks to the baking soda.

HEARTBURN AND INDIGESTION
Seaweed Stomach Soother

2 cups Irish moss – *Chondrus crispus* seaweed (see Resources on page 218)
4 tbsp fennel seeds
4 tbsp mint leaves
2 cups (500 ml) water
⅔ cup (25 ml) glycerin
4 tbsp baking soda

1 Simmer the Irish moss, fennel seeds, and mint leaves in the water for 20 to 30 minutes, or until the liquid has reduced to 1 cup (250 ml).

2 Mix in a blender with the glycerin until smooth, then strain through a sieve covered with cheesecloth. Leave to cool.

3 Whisk in the baking soda, then pour the mixture through a funnel into a sterilized bottle.

USE Take 2 tsp whenever you feel symptoms coming on. See your doctor if symptoms persist for more than a few days.

STORAGE Keeps for 1 month in the refrigerator.

A tasty liqueur that helps with all kinds of digestive problems, including colic, menstrual pain, and chills.

DIGESTION
Angelica Tummy Soother

100 g fresh angelica root, chopped
25 g fresh peppermint leaves
125 g fresh juniper berries
3 cups (750 ml) vodka
sugar to taste

1 Put the angelica, peppermint, juniper berries, and vodka into a wide-necked bottle or jar with an airtight lid or stopper. Allow to stand in sunlight or in a warm place for 10 days.

2 Strain through cheesecloth and add sugar to taste. Filter into a sterilized bottle or jar.

USE Take a small glassful 1 or 2 times a day when needed.
NOTE: This mixture contains alcohol, so be careful not to overuse, especially if driving. Do not use if pregnant.

STORAGE Keeps well for up to 6 months.

Menthol, found in mint leaves, is used in commercial preparations to treat IBS (Irritable Bowel Syndrome). An alternate way to ingest it is by simply making a cup of mint tea. This tea can also alleviate flatulence, colic, indigestion, and heartburn.

IRRITABLE BOWEL SYNDROME

Peppermint Tea

1 tbsp fresh peppermint leaves
1 drinking cup boiling water

Steep the leaves in hot water for 5 minutes.
Drink as needed.

Senna (**Senna alexandrina**), a native of the tropics, has been used for centuries as a safe and highly effective laxative. Use dried pods for this syrup, because they seem to have a gentler effect than the leaves. Adding figs provides soluble fiber to help digestion and soothe the stomach. This syrup will quickly relieve the discomfort of constipation. It is best taken before bed, since it takes 8 to 12 hours to take effect.

CONSTIPATION
Syrup of Figs

18 g dried senna pods (see Resources on page 218)
⅔ cup (100 ml) boiling water
8 fresh figs, quartered
8 tbsp (100 g) sugar
juice of 1 lemon

1 Place the senna pods in a glass bowl and cover with the boiling water. Leave to steep for about 30 minutes, then strain through a sieve or piece of cheesecloth into a blender.

2 Add the figs and sugar to the senna infusion and blend until smooth.

3 Pour into a saucepan, and heat slowly to reduce, stirring occasionally. You want to end up with a thick, glossy sugarlike syrup; this will probably take about 25 minutes. Add the lemon juice and stir in well.

4 Remove from the heat and pour the syrup into a small sterilized bottle.

USE Shake well before use. Take 2 tsp before bed as needed.
NOTE: Don't use for more than a few days at a time. Discontinue using if you have severe abdominal pain.

STORAGE Keeps in the refrigerator for 3 to 4 weeks.

VARIATION
Senna and Ginger Tea

Take 1 tsp dried senna pods, add a little less than an inch (2 cm) gingerroot, peeled and chopped, and pour over 1 cup (250 ml) freshly boiled water. Leave for 10 minutes to infuse. Strain. Add lemon juice if desired. Drink while still warm, before bedtime.

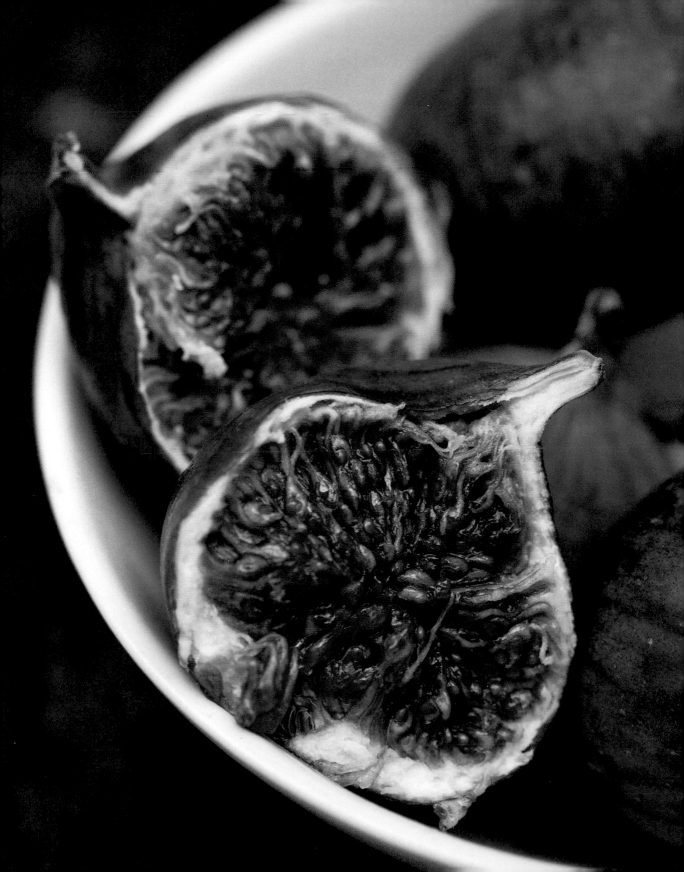

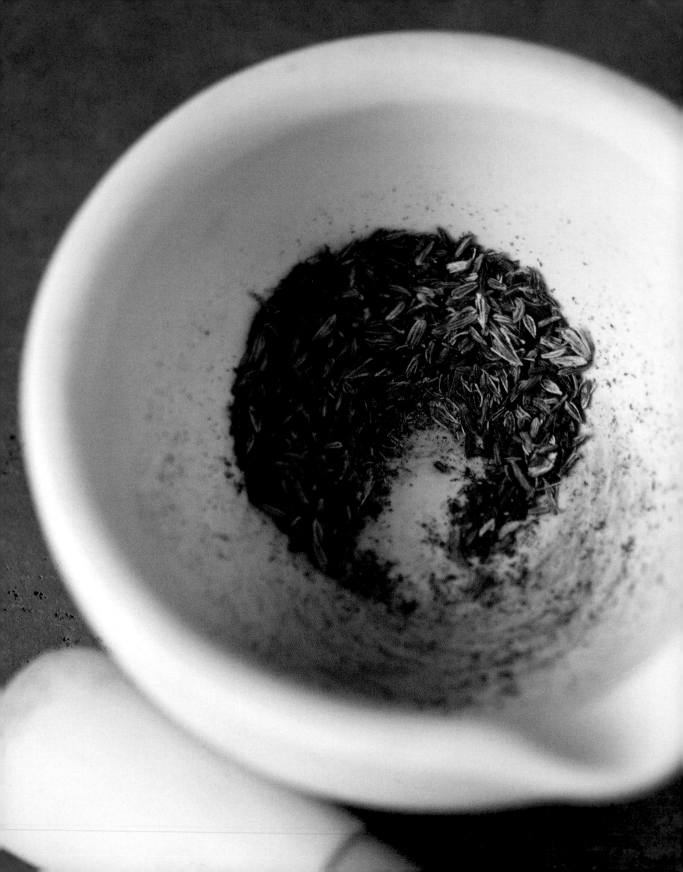

A fresh, tangy brew with four ingredients that all work to release trapped intestinal gas—which may explain its name. The herbs have an antispasmodic effect that relaxes the stomach, so gas can escape and bloating can be relieved.

FLATULENCE
"Four Winds" Tea

1 tsp caraway seeds
1 tsp fennel seeds
1 tsp chopped peppermint leaves
1 tsp chamomile flowers
1 cup (250 ml) boiling water

1 Crush the caraway and fennel seeds in a mortar and pestle to help extract the oils. Combine the seeds with the peppermint and chamomile. Place in an airtight container.

2 To make the tea, put 1 to 2 tsp of the mix in 1 cup (250 ml) hot (not boiling) water and allow the herbs to infuse for about 15 minutes. Sip slowly, while still warm.

USE Drink a cup when needed, up to 4 times a day.

STORAGE The herb mixture keeps very well in an airtight container for several months. Make the tea fresh before drinking.

Diarrhea quickly drains the body of fluids, salts, and other minerals. This recipe, which uses the World Health Organization formula for rehydration salts in the form of a stomach-soothing herbal tea, replaces electrolyte salts quickly and effectively. Take a container of the tea mixture with you whenever you're traveling.

DIARRHEA
Herbal Rehydration Tea

½ tsp salt
¼ tsp potassium chloride ("low sodium" salt)
¼ tsp baking soda
2 tbsp glucose
½–1 tbsp fennel seeds
½–1 tbsp peppermint leaves
1 qt (1 L) water, boiled just before use

1 In a bowl, combine the salts, glucose, and herbs, and mix well.

2 Add the water (just boiled but not boiling) and allow the herbs to infuse for about 15 minutes. The seeds and leaves will sink to the bottom. Drink as much as possible to replace depleted electrolytes.

STORAGE The salt-and-herb mixture keeps very well in an airtight container for several months. Make the tea fresh before drinking.

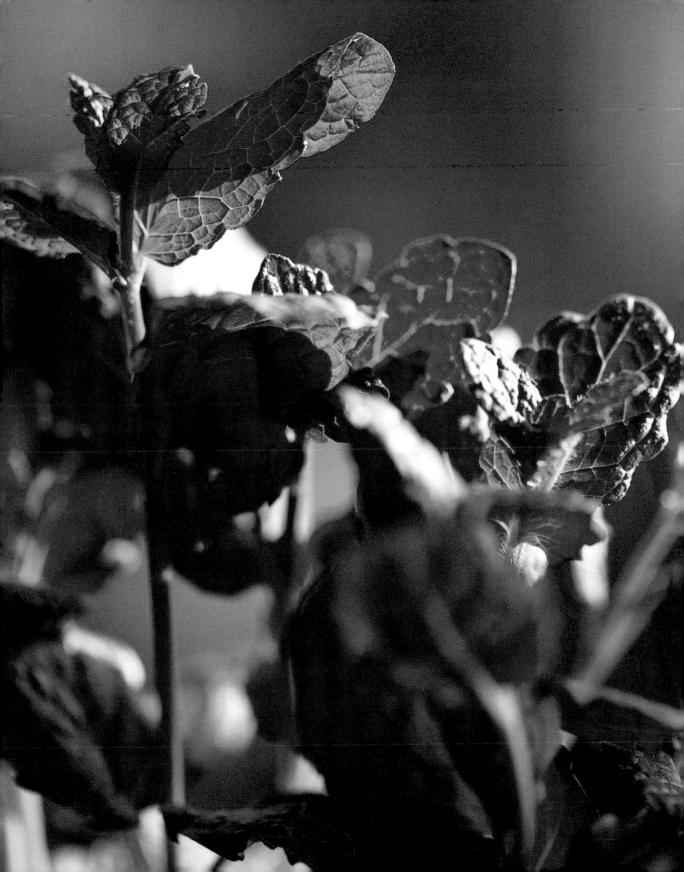

SKIN COMPLAINTS

Athlete's foot (*Tinea pedis*) is an irritating and sometimes painful fungal infection that thrives in the moist, dark areas between the toes. This powder keeps feet dry, and the garlic and tea tree oil have potent antifungal properties, which also helps to beat foot odor. For a double hit, use in conjunction with "Garlic Footbath" on page 55.

ATHLETE'S FOOT
Garlic Talcum Powder

4 tbsp dried sage leaves
4 tbsp dried garlic (commercially prepared is fine)
7 tbsp (70 g) cornstarch
7 tbsp (70 g) baking soda
24 drops tea tree essential oil

1 Grind the dried sage in a mortar and pestle, then place in a medium-sized bowl. Add the dried garlic. Sprinkle the cornstarch and baking soda on top and mix well.

2 Add in the tea tree oil and stir until well distributed. Place the powder into a salt or sugar shaker for easy use.

USE Dust on liberally 3 times daily, until symptoms disappear (usually within a few weeks). Continue using for 1 week after all signs of infection have disappeared, since previously dormant fungal spores can cause reinfection.

STORAGE Keep in a dry, dark place and use within 1 year.

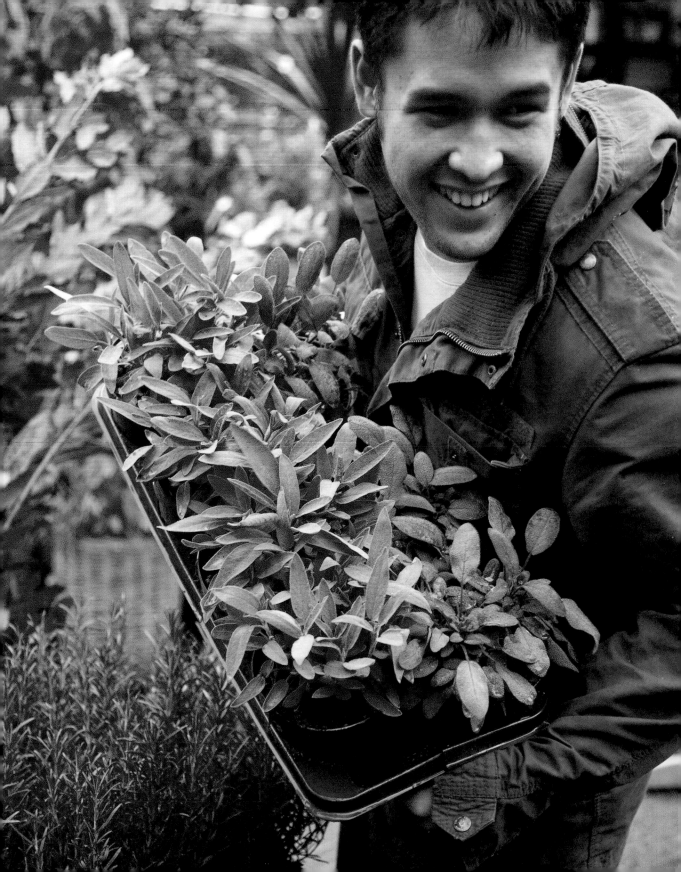

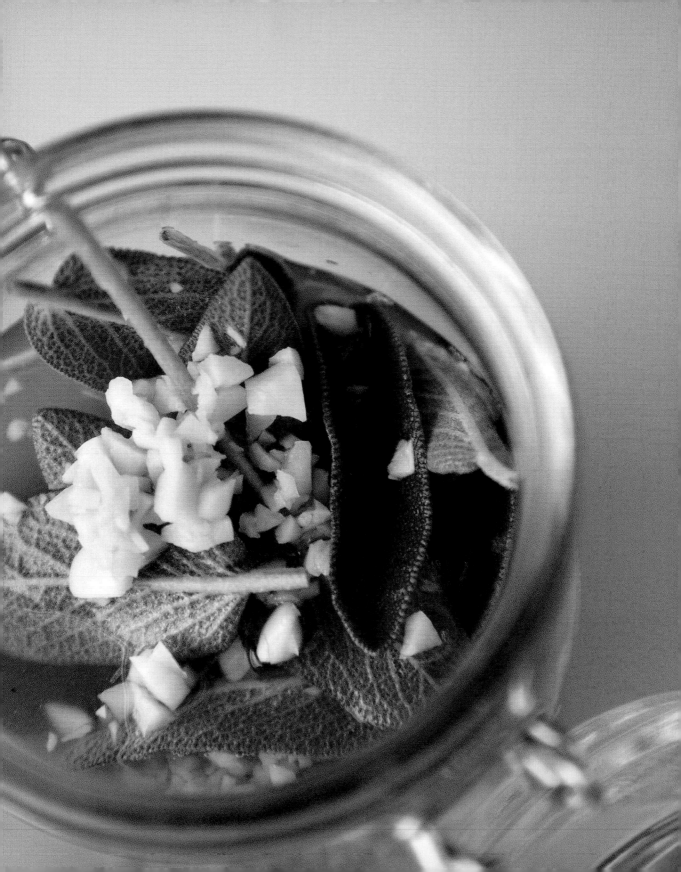

A few tablespoons of this garlicky vinegar in hot water make a powerful antifungal foot bath, but don't use it on broken skin—it will hurt! The vinegar takes 1 month to infuse but will last at least 6 months to 1 year. It tastes good in salad dressings, too.

ATHLETE'S FOOT
Garlic Footbath

10 bulbs garlic, peeled and finely chopped
100 g fresh sage leaves
2 cups (500 ml) cider vinegar

1 Place the chopped garlic and sage leaves in a jar, then add the cider vinegar. Seal and leave to infuse for 1 month, shaking occasionally.

USE Add 5 tbsp to a bowl of hot water, and soak feet for 15 minutes. Use 2 or 3 times a week in conjunction with "Garlic Talcum Powder" (see page 52).

The flowers of **Viola tricolor** have been used for centuries as an anti-inflammatory to treat skin conditions. Combined with the antihistamine and antiseptic properties of chamomile, this recipe makes a soothing balm for eczema.

ECZEMA
Viola and Chamomile Cream

Makes one 150-ml pot
2 tbsp (20 g) Johnny-jump-up flowers, stripped from their stems
2 tbsp (20 g) Roman or German chamomile, dried
1 cup (250 ml) freshly boiled water
1 tsp beeswax
2 tbsp almond oil
1 tsp vitamin C powder
1 tsp glycerin
2 tsp emulsifying wax

1 Place the Johnny-jump-ups and chamomile flowers in a glass bowl. Add the water to cover. Let infuse for 10 minutes.

2 In the top of a double boiler, add the beeswax, almond oil, vitamin C powder, glycerin, and emulsifying wax. Warm over a gentle heat, stirring until melted, about 10 minutes.

3 Strain the infusion, then slowly whisk it into the beeswax oil mixture until incorporated—the texture should be smooth, like mayonnaise.

4 Pour the mixture into a sterilized dark glass ointment jar, then seal.

USE Apply to affected areas morning and night. Ideally, apply within a few minutes after bathing to keep moisture in the skin.

STORAGE Keeps for up to 6 months in the refrigerator.

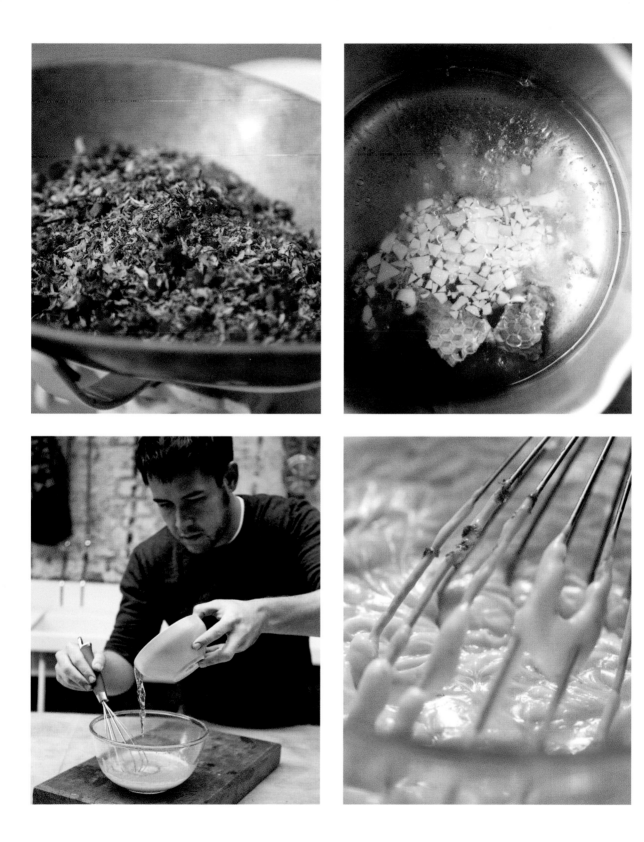

Insect bites cause immediate redness, swelling, and itching. Take the heat out of them with plantain, which has both anti-inflammatory and antiallergenic properties.

INSECT BITES AND STINGS
Plantain Cream

4 tbsp fresh plantain leaves
⅔ cup (150 ml) boiling water
2 tbsp olive oil or sunflower oil
2 tbsp almond oil
1 tsp beeswax
2 tsp emulsifying wax
2 tsp glycerin
1 tsp vitamin C powder

1 Wash and chop the plantain leaves. Divide into two—put one half in a bowl and the other half in a pan. Cover the plantain in the bowl with the water and leave to infuse for 10 minutes.

2 In the pan, add the olive (or sunflower) and almond oils to the plantain and heat gently to simmer. Remove from heat and leave for 10 minutes to cool.
NOTE: Do not boil—if mixture starts to boil, remove from heat immediately.

3 Drain the infusion, and remove the plantain leaves. Set the liquid aside.

4 Drain the infused oil into another pan, extracting the plantain leaves. Heat the oil again. Add the beeswax and emulsifying wax and melt, stirring. Aim for a foamy consistency.

5 Add 1 cup infused water to the pan and whisk to achieve a consistency like salad dressing. Add the glycerin and vitamin C powder.

6 Pour into sterilized glass jars and seal.

USE Apply to affected area as often as needed.

STORAGE Keeps for 3 months in the refrigerator in an airtight container.

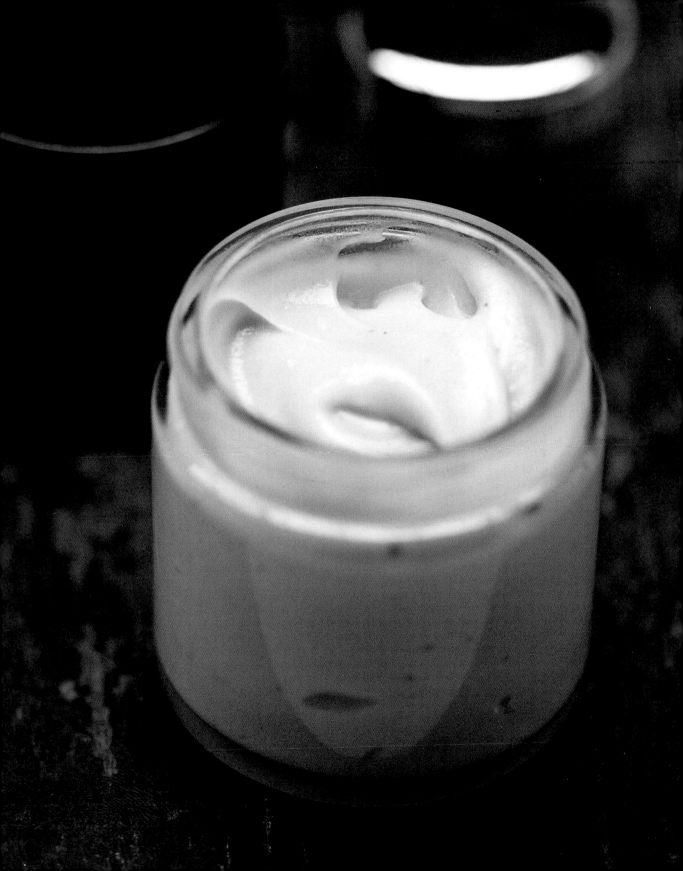

Native Americans traditionally used the leaves, bark, and twigs of witch hazel (*Hamamelis virginiana*) as a skin compress. Its astringent, antibacterial properties make it especially useful for blemishes and skin irritations. This gel is gentler than many over-the-counter blemish ointments, which can leave your skin dry and flaky. Carry a jar with you and use whenever needed.

BLEMISHES
Witch Hazel Gel

200 g witch hazel twigs and (preferably young) leaves
   (see Resources on page 218)
2 cups (500 ml) hot water
6 packets vegetable gelatin
2 tbsp vodka

1 Place the witch hazel in a pan with the hot water. Over a gentle heat, slowly reduce mixture to a third of its volume until it reaches about ⅔ cup of liquid (this will take about 1 hour).

2 Line a sieve with cheesecloth, then strain the liquid into a mixing bowl. Add the gelatin, stirring to dissolve. Set aside to cool.

3 Once cool, add the vodka and stir well. Pour the gel into a wide-mouthed jar.

USE Dab on blemishes and skin irritations whenever needed.

STORAGE Keeps for up to 6 months in the refrigerator.

The gel from the fleshy leaves of the aloe vera plant is ideal for soothing and speeding the healing of sunburn and other minor wounds. This gentle preparation, applied topically, can be used on children, too.

SUNBURN
Carrot and Aloe Cream

2 carrots
1 cucumber
½ cup sesame oil
1 tsp beeswax
2 tsp emulsifying wax
½ cup aloe vera gel
1 tsp vitamin C powder

1 Finely grate the carrot and cucumber and place in a large pan with the sesame oil. Heat very gently for 20 to 30 minutes. Strain, then return the liquid to the pan.

2 Add the beeswax and emulsifying wax to the pan, and stir while they melt. Whisk in the aloe vera and vitamin C powder. Keep whisking until the mixture becomes creamy and smooth.

3 Pour into a wide-mouthed jar, and let cool. The cream will thicken while cooling.

USE Apply liberally to any sunburned or sore areas 2 or 3 times a day.

STORAGE Keeps for up to 2 months in the refrigerator.

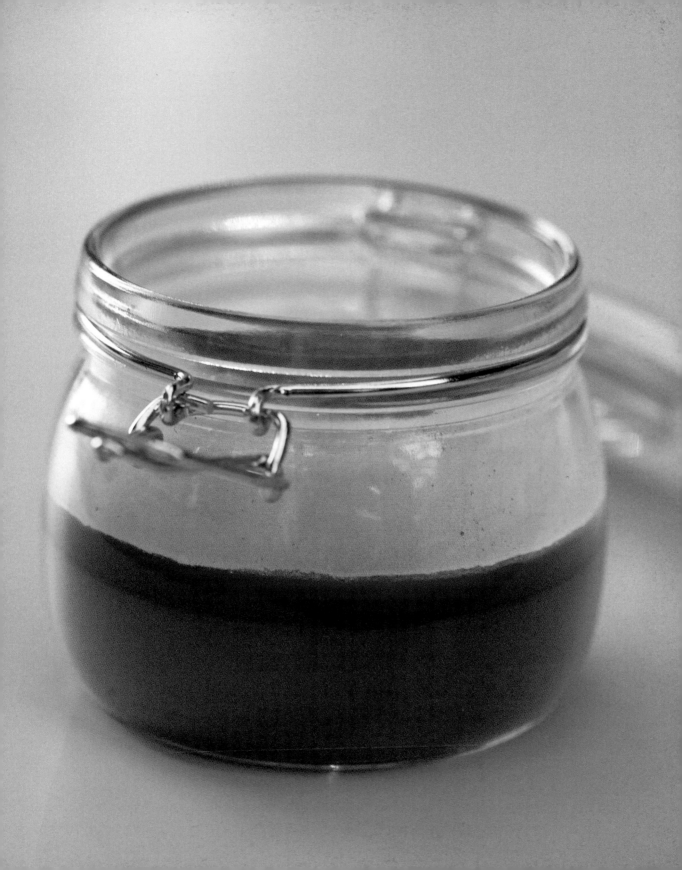

Bright orange marigolds (*Calendula officinalis*) contain salicylic acid—used in many over-the-counter acne treatments—plus anti-inflammatory and antiseptic substances, which make it a favorite for skin conditions of many kinds. If used over a period of weeks, this gel should significantly alleviate the appearance of acne and reduce discomfort.

ACNE

Marigold, Lavender, and Rose Geranium Gel

10 rose geranium flowers, with leaves and stems
8 marigold (*Calendula officinalis*) flowers
20 lavender flowerheads
¾ cup (200 ml) water
1 packet vegetable gelatin
5 tsp vodka
20 drops tea tree oil

1 Roughly chop the flowers, leaves, and stems of the rose geraniums and place with the marigold flowers and lavender flowerheads in a large glass bowl.

2 Bring the water to a boil and pour it over the flowers to make an infusion. Leave to infuse for 10 minutes or until the water has taken on the color of the flowers. Place the infusion, including the plant material, into a blender and mix. Strain the mixture through a piece of cheesecloth into a clean bowl.

3 In another bowl, dissolve the gelatin in 2 tbsp cold water. Gradually add the flower infusion, stirring to separate lumps. Add the vodka and tea tree oil, stirring until a gel is formed. Using a funnel, pour into a jar with a pump dispenser.

USE Apply to affected areas twice a day or as frequently as needed.

STORAGE Keeps in the refrigerator for up to 6 weeks.

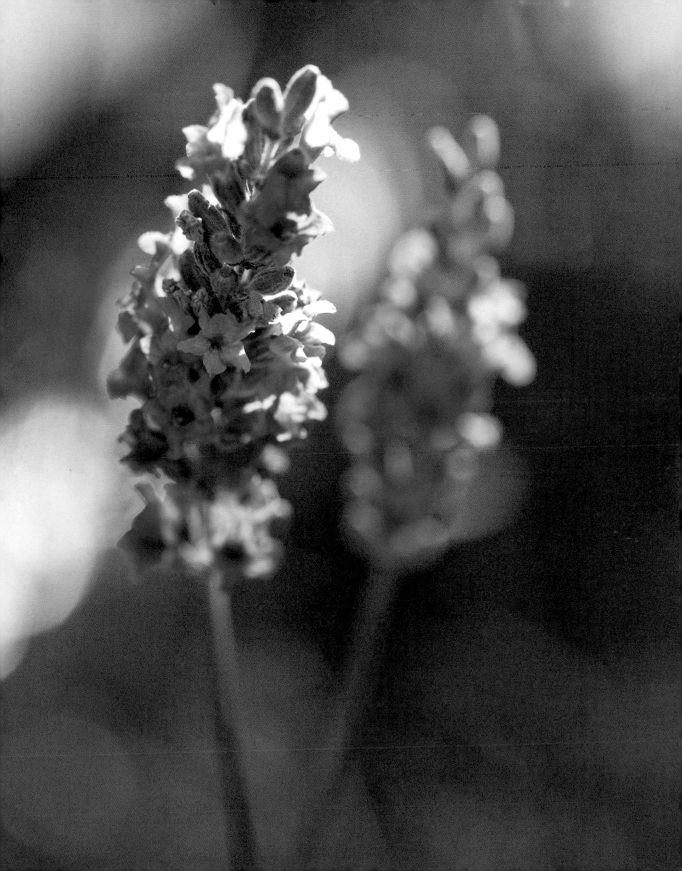

This soap is excellent for ringworm, athlete's foot, and thrush. It also makes a good antiseptic hand wash because both tea tree and thyme are potent antifungals. Soap molds may be bought online.

FUNGAL SKIN CONDITIONS

Antiseptic Soap

300 g white soap
2 cups (500 ml) water
5 tbsp almond oil (or olive, jojoba, or avocado oil)
2 tsp tea tree essential oil
30 drops thyme (*Thymus vulgaris,* ct. linalool) essential oil
4 tbsp dried marigold (*Calendula officinalis*) flowers

1 Grate the white soap into a glass bowl, then add the water. Place the bowl over a pan of boiling water on low heat. Stir continuously until the soap melts.

2 Add the almond oil and tea tree and thyme oils. Then add the dried flowers, mixing well with a metal spoon.

3 Pour the mixture into a shallow dish to make a soap "loaf," or into individual soap molds. Leave to cool and set; this may take up to 1 week.

4 Once set, cut the soap loaf into shapes or turn out of the molds. Wrap the soaps in wax paper and let dry in a cool place until needed.

USE Wash affected areas with the soap once or twice daily, or as required. Rinse well after using.

STORAGE Store, wrapped in wax paper, in a cool, dark place. Keeps for up to 1 year.

Juniper (*Juniperus communis*) contains powerful anti-inflammatory and astringent substances. You may make just the oil and use it to massage the body to stimulate circulation and relieve back pain. Or you may choose to add beeswax to the oil to create a healing ointment that can soothe itching, and scratches.

HEALING OINTMENT
Juniper Oil

125 g fresh juniper berries (preferably just ripening)
1 cup (250 ml) olive or sunflower oil
3 or 4 tbsp beeswax (for ointment only)

To make the massage oil:

1 Soak the berries in water overnight to soften, then strain and discard the water.

2 Place the berries in a double boiler, then add the oil and simmer gently, taking care not to burn, for 30 minutes, or until the berries lose their color and the oil darkens.

3 Strain through a sieve lined with cheesecloth, reserving the oil. Pour into a sterilized glass bottle to store.

USE Massage well into the affected area 2 or 3 times a day.

STORAGE Keeps for at least 6 months.

To make the healing ointment:

Make the "Juniper Oil" as described. Heat the beeswax in a double boiler over low heat. Add the oil to the double boiler, mixing thoroughly. Pour into a sterilized dark glass jar. As the mixture cools, the balm will solidify. If the ointment is too soft, remove from the pot and add a little more melted wax. Gently reheat the mixture until smooth, then bottle as before.

USE Apply 2 or 3 times a day to affected area.

STORAGE Keeps for 6 months in a sterilized dark glass jar.

Remedies: Skin Complaints

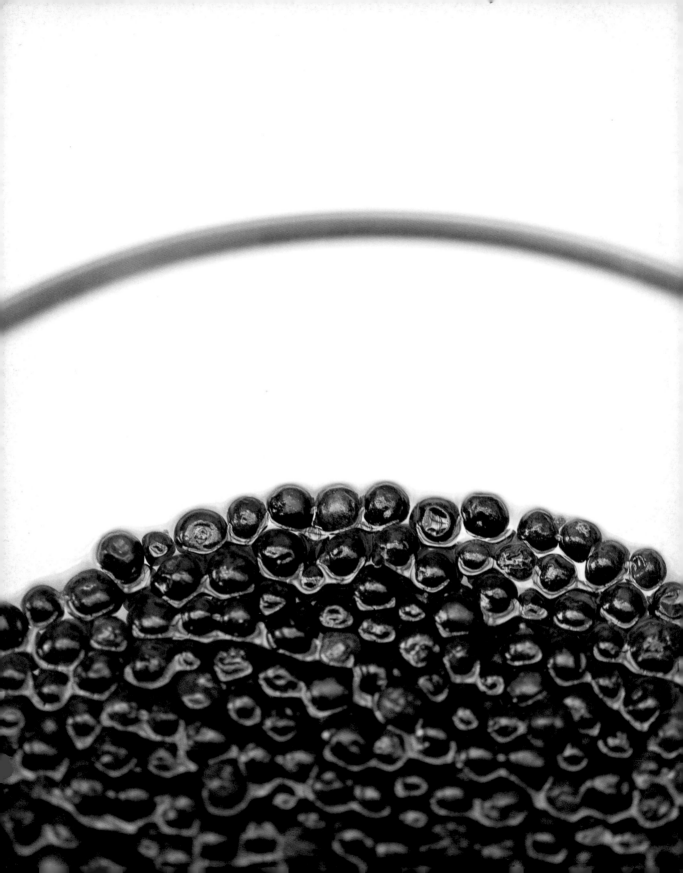

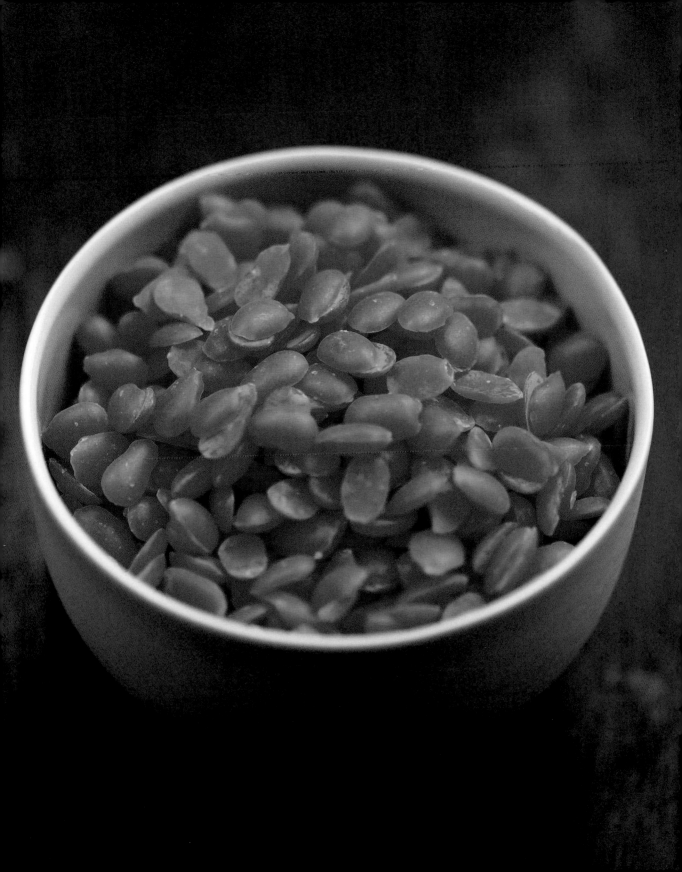

This hot oil will make the blood race to your feet. Apply every day before bed to improve circulation and to help prevent cold feet and chilblains.

COLD FEET
Hot Chili and Mustard Foot Oil

2 cups (500 ml) sunflower oil
2–4 fresh whole red chilies (cayenne), chopped
50 g gingerroot, chopped or crushed
50 g black pepper
50 g mustard powder

1 In the top of a double boiler, place the sunflower oil, chopped chilies, gingerroot, black pepper, and mustard powder. Stir to mix. Heat the mixture gently for 1 hour.

2 Strain through a sieve lined with cheesecloth. Filter the oil into sterilized dark glass bottles.

USE Rub a little of the oil directly into the feet at night to encourage circulation.
NOTE: This oil does heat the skin, so wash your hands after use; keep away from eyes and other sensitive areas.

STORAGE Keeps for up to 6 months.

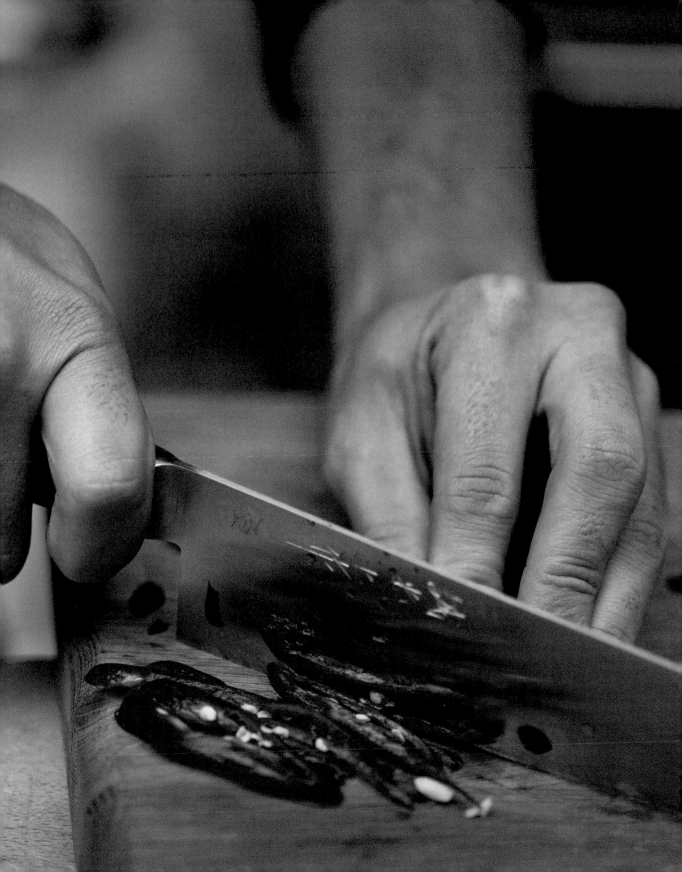

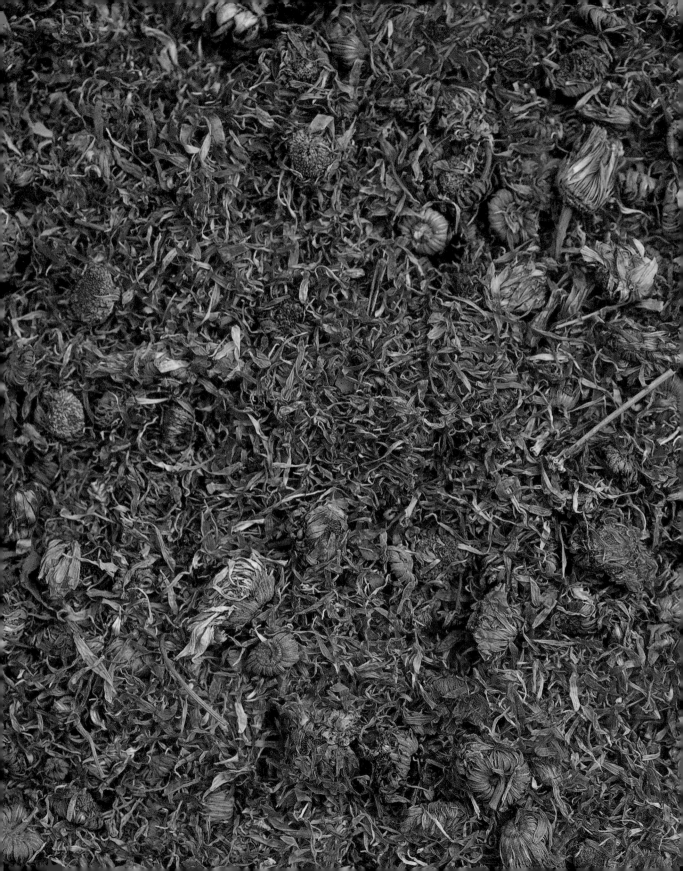

This gentle salve for chapped hands, skin inflammations, wounds, and hemorrhoids is very easy to make. Eucalyptus has a powerful aroma that you either love or hate—you may leave it out if you wish.

CHAPPED HANDS AND SORES
Jelly Balm

25 g St.-John's-wort flowers
20 g marigold (*Calendula officinalis*) flowers
olive oil, to cover
white petroleum jelly—2 parts to 1 part of oil
eucalyptus essential oil (optional)

1 Put the St.-John's-wort and marigold flowers in a jar and cover with the olive oil. Allow to stand in a cool place for 1 week and then strain through cheesecloth.

2 Melt the petroleum jelly using a double boiler. Add 1 part of the oil made above to 2 parts of melted petroleum jelly. Stir while cooling—you can also add a few drops of eucalyptus oil at this stage if you like. Pour into a sterilized glass jar before the ointment solidifies.

USE Gently rub into the affected area 3 or 4 times a day when needed.

STORAGE Keeps for at least 6 months in the refrigerator.

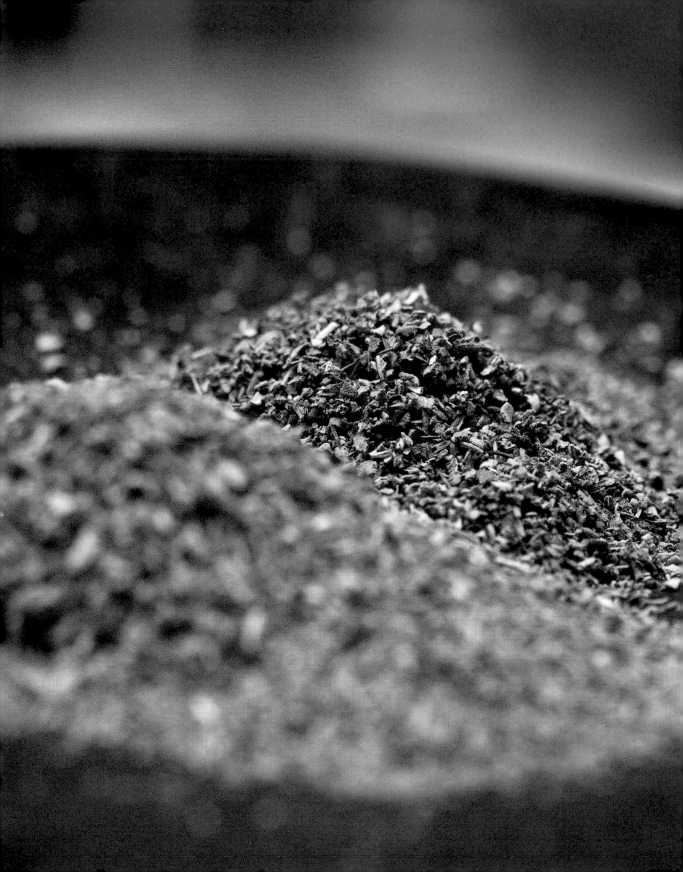

This recipe provides a very simple way to deter flying pests and protect yourself from bites and stings. Sage, rosemary, and wormwood are well known as insect repellents, containing camphor and other essential oils. You can use store-bought dried herbs, although drying your own fresh leaves will produce a more aromatic mix.

INSECT DETERRENT
Pest Potpourri

2 tbsp dried rosemary leaves
2 tbsp dried wormwood leaves (see Resources on page 218)
2 tbsp dried sage leaves

Strip the leaves from the plants, and crush them finely. Mix together in a shallow bowl, and leave in a warm place to encourage the oils to vaporize.

STORAGE Keeps for at least 1 month, or until the aroma has evaporated.

KIDS

Rosehip syrup is an old-fashioned winter remedy for boosting vitamin levels and keeping colds at bay. Gather the hips in October and November when they're ripe and soft. Children love this syrup, and it's good poured over pancakes, waffles, ice cream, and rice pudding.

VITAMIN BOOSTER
Vitamin C–Rich Rosehip Syrup

250 g fresh rosehips (see Resources on page 218)
5 cloves (optional)
1 cinnamon stick (optional)
2 cups (500 ml) water
about ½ cup (125 g) sugar

1 Crush the rosehips slightly, and place in a pan. Add the cloves and cinnamon stick, if using, then add the water. Simmer, uncovered, for 20 minutes.

2 Strain, then add the same amount of sugar as there is liquid. Stir until dissolved and bring to a boil, then simmer for 10 minutes. Cool and filter into small sterilized bottles.

USE For children, give 2 tsp per day. To drink as a cordial, dilute 1 part syrup to 5 parts water. Or use instead of maple syrup for the dishes suggested above.

STORAGE Keeps for 1 week in the refrigerator once opened. Unopened, keeps for up to 1 year.

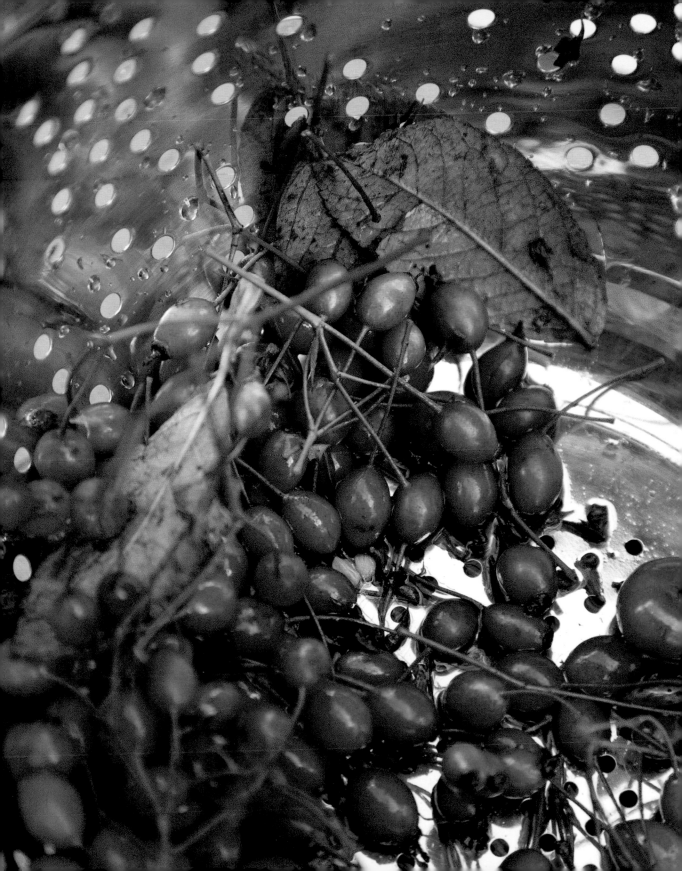

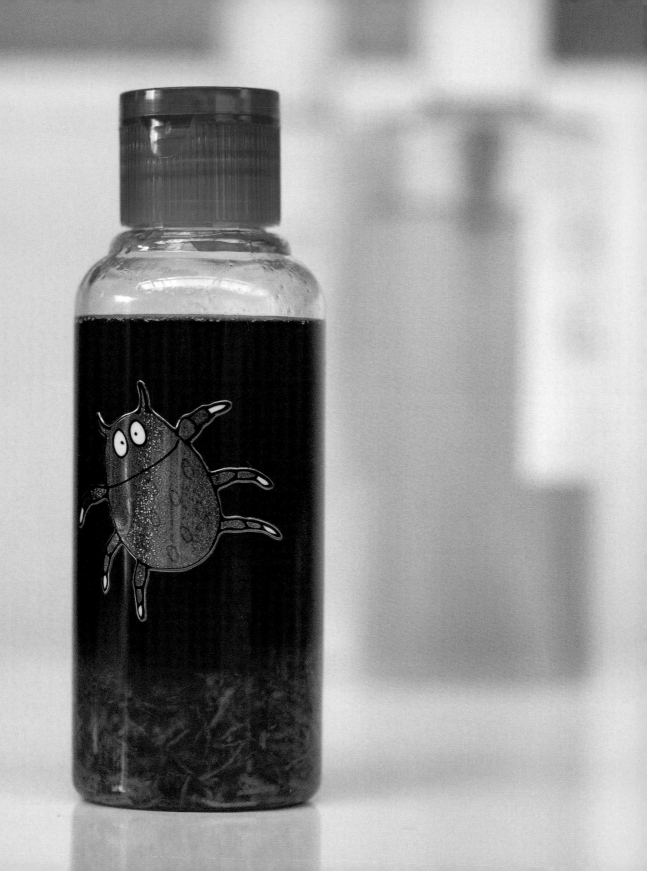

With up to 80 percent of head lice now resistant to conventional treatments, the hunt is on for an effective and safe insecticide to treat nits—the tiny eggs that are notoriously hard to eradicate. This natural recipe, free of organophosphates, uses plant extracts with known insecticidal properties to kill both lice and the nits.

HEAD LICE

Neem Nit Treatment
Makes enough for 5–10 doses

20 tbsp (approx. 100 g) fresh rosemary leaves
20 tbsp (approx. 25 g) fresh lavender flowers
¾ cup (200 ml) neem oil
¾ cup (200 ml) almond oil
6 garlic cloves, minced
2 tbsp tea tree essential oil

1 Strip the rosemary leaves and lavender flowers from their sprigs.

2 Combine the neem and almond oil together in a measuring cup.

3 Crush half the rosemary and lavender in a mortar and pestle with a little of the oil to help ease the crushing process. Place the mashed-up herbs in a saucepan. Repeat with the second half of the rosemary and lavender, again adding a little oil for crushing.

4 Place the crushed herbs and the neem and almond oil in the pan, and add the minced garlic. Heat gently for about 20 minutes.

5 Strain through a sieve lined with cheesecloth. Add the tea tree oil to the reserved oil, stir, then filter into a sterilized ½ pint (500 ml) bottle.

USE If using immediately, apply to dry hair, making sure that the hair is completely covered and that the oil penetrates to the scalp. Cover with a towel and leave on for at least 1 hour, or overnight if possible. Then wash off with two applications of shampoo. Apply conditioner, and comb through with a nit comb. Use the next application 7 days later, to deal with any nits that may hatch during that time. Comb through with the nit comb every 3 days.

STORAGE Keeps for 6 months.

A wonderful way to introduce herbs to children is simply by adding them to their bathwater. This infusion—made with Roman chamomile instead of German—soothes eczema, the red, itchy, inflamed skin condition that is common in babies and children. The flowerheads bob around like pom-poms and are fun for children to play with.

ECZEMA
Pom-Pom Bath

4 handfuls (approx. 40 g) Roman chamomile
   (*Chamaemelum nobile*) flowerheads
1 qt (1 L) freshly boiled water

Place the chamomile in a glass bowl, then add the freshly boiled water and let stand, covered, for about 15 minutes.

USE Add straight to bathwater. Alternatively, strain the flowerheads and discard.

STORAGE Make fresh each time before using.

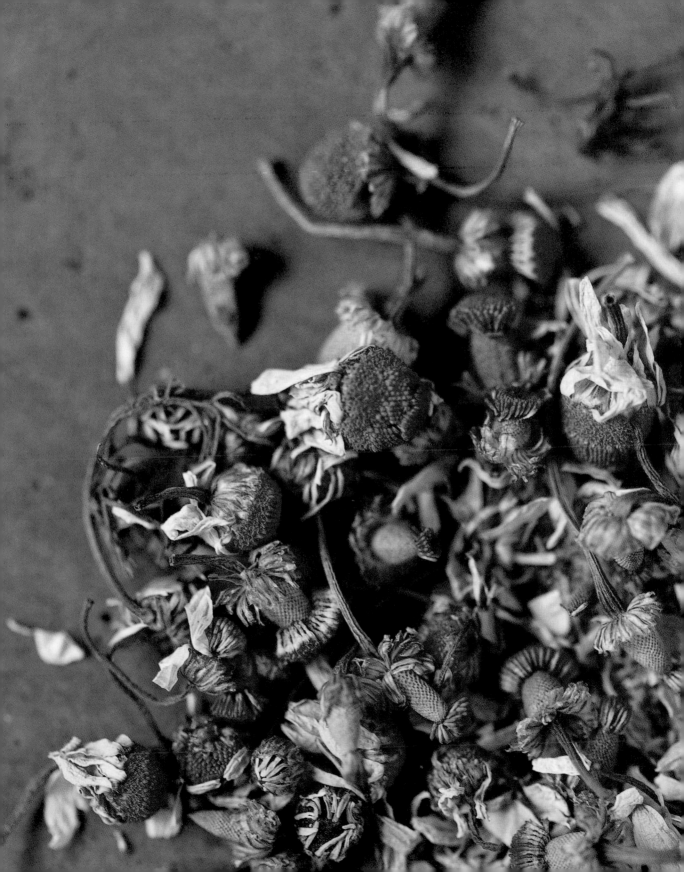

A simple remedy containing mullein (***Verbascum thapsus***)—traditionally used to soothe inflammation and aid healing—and almond oil to soften wax.

EARWAX BUILDUP
Wax-Dissolving Drops

1 small handful mullein flowers
1 cup (250 ml) almond oil

1 Cover the mullein flowers with the oil and let steep for several days in sunlight.

2 Alternatively, you can place the flowers and oil in a small pan and warm on the stove over very gentle heat for several hours.

3 Strain through cheesecloth and a small filter into sterilized dropper bottles.

USE Place a few drops into the affected ear(s) morning and night, or up to 4 times a day to relieve pain and soften wax. Continue treatment for at least 5 days.
NOTE: If pain continues or wax remains hard, call your primary-care physician.

STORAGE Keeps for 3 months.

Sweet syrups are an easy way to get children to take herbal remedies. This multitasking chamomile syrup has a calming sedative effect, relaxes the digestive tract, and has antiallergenic properties. It's good for use with colic, stomachaches, and when a child has trouble sleeping.

COLIC
Chamomile Syrup

4 handfuls (approx 40 g) German chamomile (*Matricaria recutita*) flowerheads
4 cups (900 ml) water
2 ¼ cups (450g) sugar or 1 cup (340g) honey

1 In a pan, put the chamomile in the water and bring to a boil. Turn the heat to low, then cover with a tight-fitting lid and simmer for about 20 minutes.

2 Reduce the mixture to ¾ cup (approx 200 ml) by simmering very slowly with the lid off for an additional 20 minutes.

3 Add the sugar and simmer for a few more minutes, stirring until the mixture looks like syrup. Be careful not to boil rapidly; allow it to bubble just a little.

4 Strain through a mesh sieve and then pour it into a sterilized bottle. Seal with a cork; if the syrup ferments, the bottle might explode.

USE For a child, 1 tsp, 3 to 6 times a day. For adults, 2 to 4 tsp, 3 to 6 times a day. Caution: If you are diabetic, do not use.

STORAGE Keeps unopened for up to 1 year. Once opened, keeps for 1 week in the refrigerator.

ACHES AND PAINS

If you are prone to swollen ankles and feet, you know that the pain usually increases as the day progresses. This mixture uses plantain, dandelion, and nettle, three common garden weeds, which are all mild diuretics and traditionally used to ease symptoms caused by water retention. The dandelion restores potassium levels, which can be flushed out by many diuretics.

WATER RETENTION
Plantain Tea for Swollen Ankles

2 tbsp fresh plantain leaves
2 tbsp fresh dandelion leaves (or flowers)
2 tbsp nettle leaves
1 qt (1 L) water, freshly boiled

Wash the leaves, place in a bowl, then pour over the water. Let steep for 10 minutes. Strain.

USE This makes enough for about 3 cups, which can be drunk throughout the day.

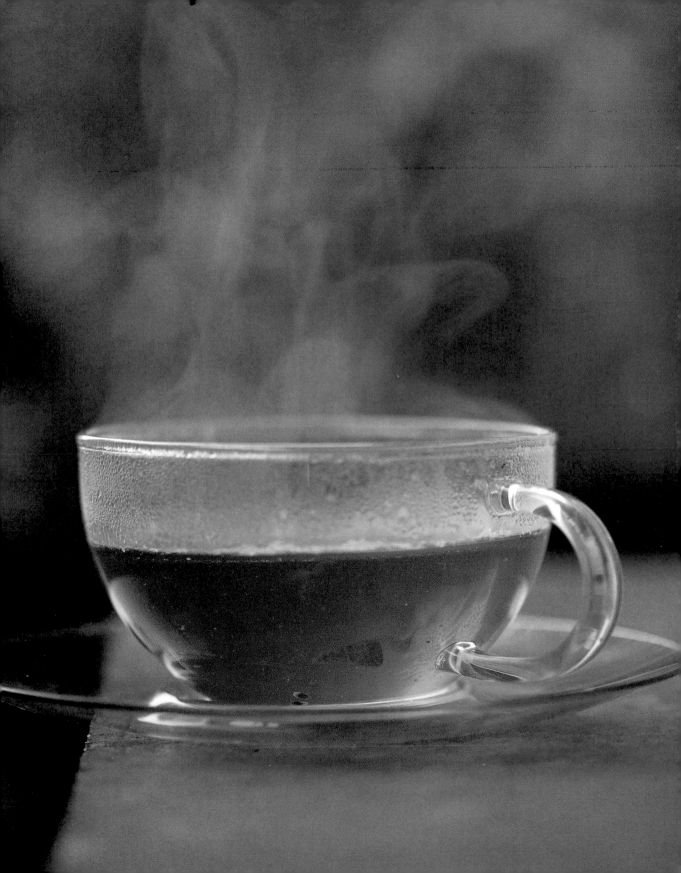

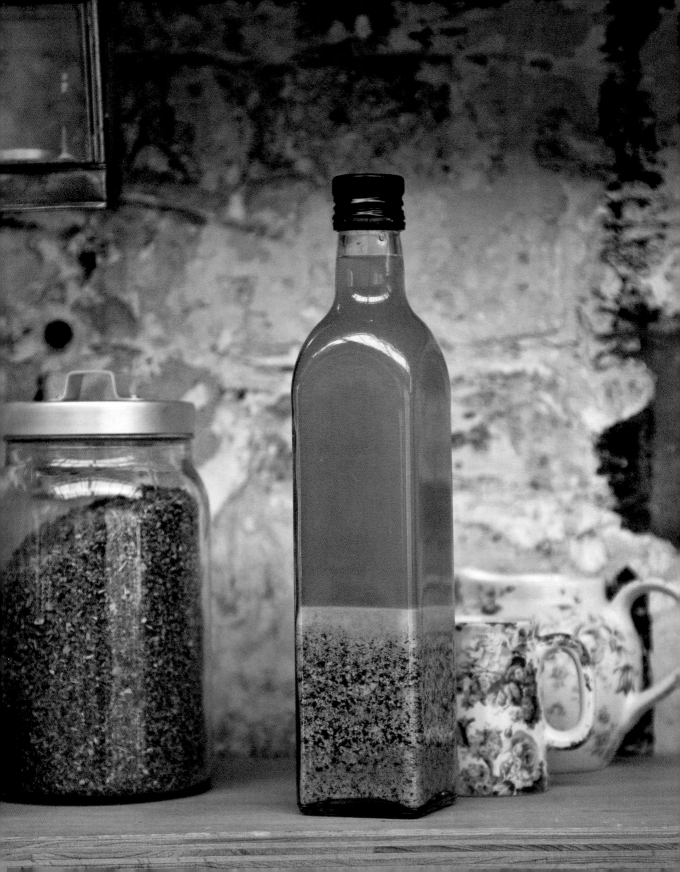

You can load up on horse chestnuts (the seeds of **Aesculus hippocastanum**) by the basketful in the fall. They contain saponins, which are frequently used in the treatment of varicose veins (and hemorrhoids) to improve the elasticity of the walls of the veins, reducing swelling and relieving the feeling of heaviness in the legs. Prepare the tincture first, then use to make the gel (see page 88).

VARICOSE VEIN GEL

Horse Chestnut Tincture

20 horse chestnuts
2 cups (500 ml) vodka

1 Place the chestnuts and vodka in a blender and mix until smooth.

2 Place in a sterilized bottle and keep in a cool, dark place for 10 days to 1 month, shaking every day or so. Strain before using.

STORAGE Keeps for up to 1 year.
CAUTION: Do not take internally. This tincture is to be used only to make the Horse Chestnut Gel (see page 88).

This slightly astringent gel feels cool and refreshing on sore, swollen legs and varicose veins. Take it with you on long flights to reduce swelling.

VARICOSE VEINS
Horse Chestnut Gel

3 packets gelatin
⅔ cup (150 ml) cold water
⅔ cup (150 ml) Horse Chestnut Tincture (see page 87)
5 drops lavender essential oil

1 In a pan, add the gelatin to the cold water and whisk until dissolved. Heat for about 2 minutes, whisking constantly. As the mixture starts to thicken, slowly pour in the Horse Chestnut Tincture a little at a time. Add the lavender oil.

2 Pour into a 1-cup (250-ml) sterilized bottle.

USE Try a 24-hour patch test on the skin before using—horse chestnuts can irritate. Apply to affected areas twice daily, or as often as required.

STORAGE The gel keeps for 3 months in the refrigerator.

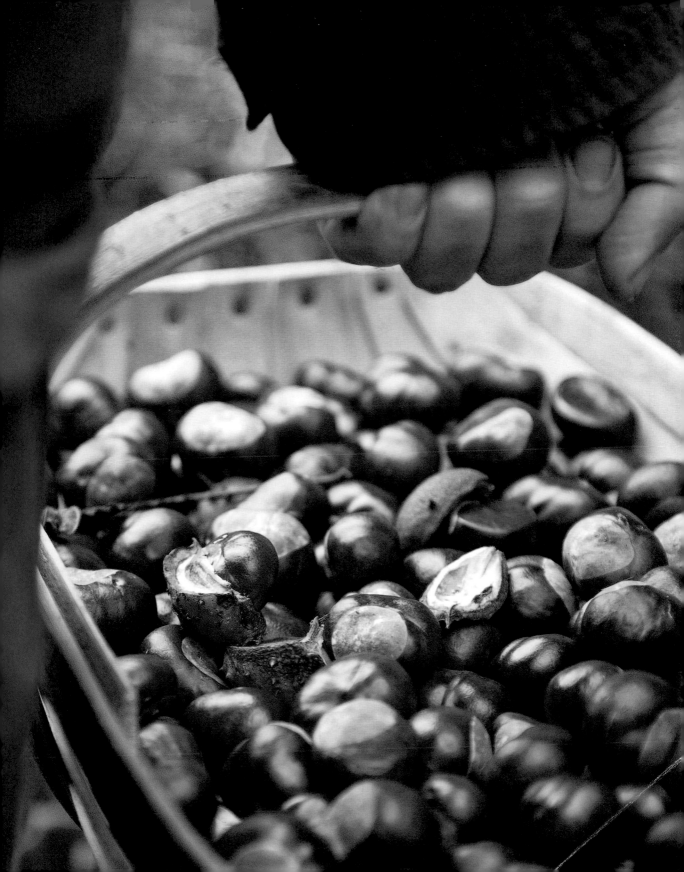

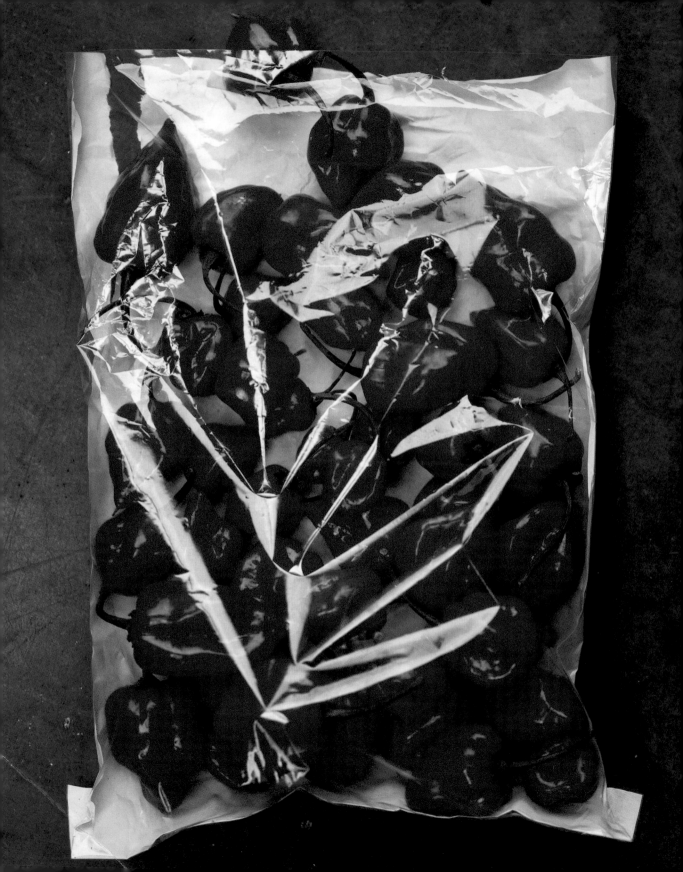

Chili and mustard work as both a local anesthetic and a deep-heat treatment to ease stiff and painful muscles. This recipe makes 4 to 5 plasters. Non-fractionated coconut oil is available in ethnic food stores. It should be white and solid at room temperature.

FOR ACHING MUSCLES
Chili Plasters

1 cup (200 g) orange Scotch Bonnet chili peppers
4 tbsp mustard powder
1 cup (200 g) coconut oil, non-fractionated
6 tsp (40 g) beeswax
4 packets gauze wound dressing pads, 4 x 4 inches (10 x 10 cm)
4 packets adhesive wound dressings, 4 x 4 inches (12 x 12 cm)

1 Wash and finely slice the chili peppers. Combine the peppers and mustard powder with the coconut oil in a saucepan. Cover and gently heat for 2 minutes. Turn off the heat and let cool with the lid on.

2 Pour the chili mixture into cheesecloth over a sieve and squeeze out the oil into a bowl underneath. Place the oil back into the saucepan and return to the heat.

3 Add the beeswax to the oil and heat very gently until dissolved; this will take less than 2 minutes. Remove from heat.

4 Soak the dressing pads in the oil mixture while it's still hot. When they are saturated, remove the pads and let stand for 10 minutes on wax paper, or until set.

5 Once set and dry, the pads can be layered on top of each other, wrapped in plastic wrap, and stored in the refrigerator until needed.

USE Place a pad on an adhesive wound dressing, then apply to the affected area. Keep the area warm (by covering with a blanket, for example) and leave on for 30 minutes to 1 hour.

STORAGE Keeps for 1 year in the refrigerator.

VARIATION
Chili Talcum Powder

Both chili powder and mustard powder can be used to make a warming "talc" that invigorates circulation. Mix together 1 tsp chili powder, 1 tsp mustard powder, and 1 tbsp cornstarch, and use this to dust cold feet before putting socks on.

To soothe the pain of both hot and cold arthritic joints,
try this spicy remedy that has been countered with peppermint
and rosemary oils for scent and pain relief.

ARTHRITIS
Chili and Peppermint Salve

¼ cup (60 ml) Hot Chili and Mustard Foot Oil
   (see page 70)
5 tsp (20 g) beeswax
30 drops peppermint essential oil
30 drops rosemary essential oil

1 Pour the oil into the top of a double boiler. Add the beeswax. Place over a pan of hot water and heat gently, stirring occasionally, until the wax melts. Take off the heat and allow to cool.

2 Just as a "skin" begins to appear on the surface of the oil, add the peppermint and rosemary oils using a dropper. Mix well. Pour the mixture into a sterilized dark glass jar. Allow to cool before putting on the lid.

USE Apply twice daily to affected areas, remembering to wash hands after use. CAUTION: This oil is hot, so keep away from eyes and other sensitive areas.

STORAGE Keeps for up to 6 months.

VARIATION
Cabbage Leaf Poultice

1 Cabbage leaf has been used for centuries for swelling, ulcers, sprains, and strains. In one Swiss hospital, patients with rheumatoid arthritis have their swollen joints wrapped at night in cabbage leaves to help reduce joint swelling and pain.

2 Savoy cabbages work best. To make your own poultice: Take some cabbage leaves, cut out the central rib, lay them flat on a chopping board, and bash with a rolling pin until the juices start to come out. Then place the leaves over the swollen joints and wrap a gauze bandage around the joint to keep the leaves in place.

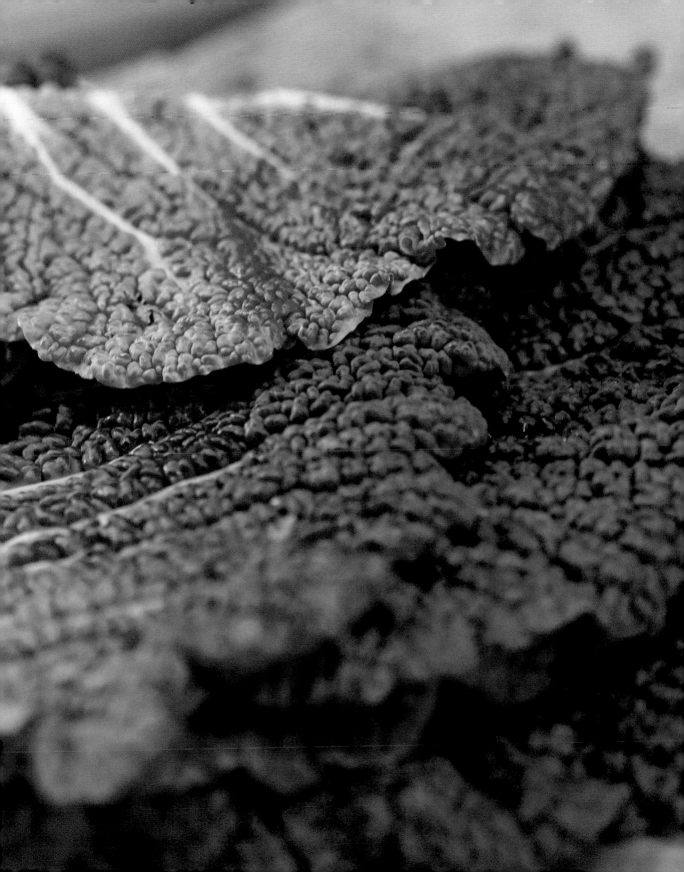

WOMEN'S STUFF

Try this simple tea for hot flushes and night sweats. No one quite knows why sage reduces sweating—possibly because of its astringency—while raspberry leaves are traditionally used to balance female hormones. Brew this tea up fresh before drinking.

HOT FLUSHES AND NIGHT SWEATS
Sage and Raspberry Leaf Tea

½ tbsp fresh sage leaves
   (if dried, use half the amount)
½ tbsp fresh raspberry leaves
   (if dried, use half the amount)
¾ cup (200 ml) freshly boiled water

Pour the water over the washed sage and raspberry leaves, and leave to infuse for 8 to 10 minutes.

USE Sip a small glassful every 3 hours.
CAUTION: Do not use if you are pregnant.

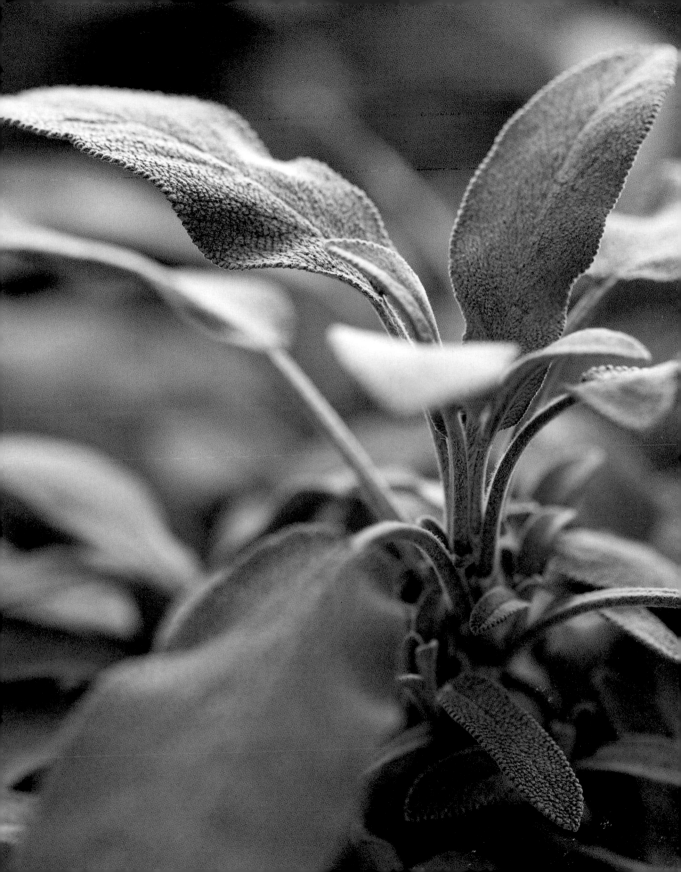

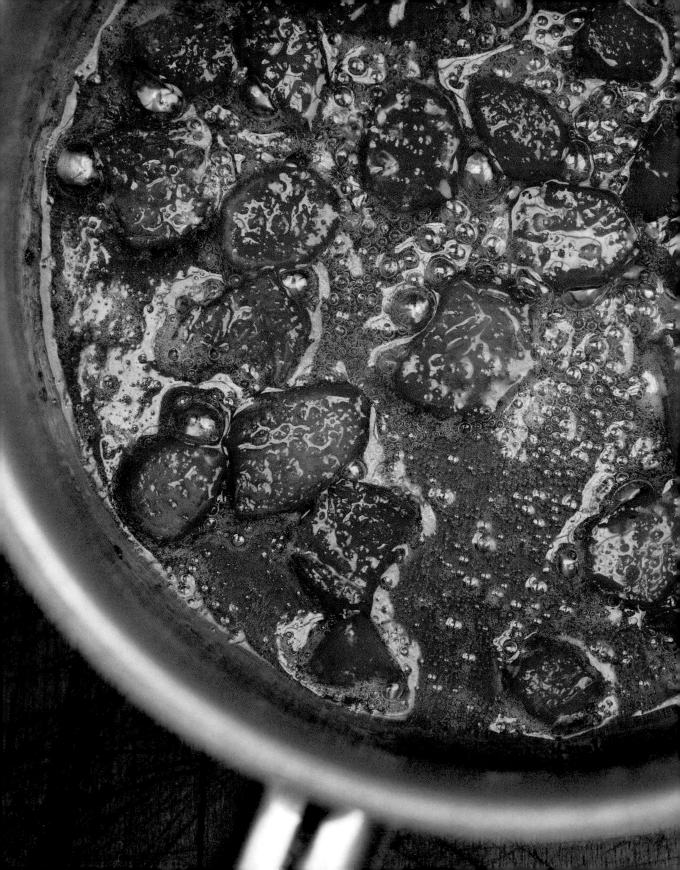

Ginger is a safe and effective treatment for both morning and motion sickness. These slices of crystallized ginger are easy to keep in a small jar in your handbag or desk and are great to chew on when you're feeling queasy.

MORNING AND MOTION SICKNESS

Crystallized Ginger
Makes about 250 g

1½ cups (350 g) fresh gingerroot
golden caster or superfine sugar, to match weight of cooked ginger,
   plus extra for sprinkling

1 Peel the fresh gingerroot and thinly slice.

2 Put the ginger in a heavy saucepan and cover with water, adding more to allow for evaporation. Bring to a boil and partly cover with a lid. Boil gently for 1 hour, or until the ginger is almost cooked but slightly al dente; the time will vary slightly depending on the freshness of the ginger.

3 Drain, remove the ginger from the pan and weigh it. Return it to the saucepan with an equal amount of sugar. Add 2 tbsp of water. Bring to a boil, then simmer over medium heat, stirring with a wooden spoon for 20 minutes, or until the ginger becomes transparent.

4 Reduce the heat and keep stirring until the ginger starts to crystallize and easily comes together or clumps in the middle of the pan.

5 Meanwhile, take a large, deep baking pan and sprinkle sugar on it. Tip the ginger into the baking pan and roll it around in the sugar. Separate any clumps of ginger pieces. Place in a sterilized jar.

USE Chew on a piece of crystallized ginger whenever you feel nauseous.

STORAGE Keeps in a cool place for 3 to 6 months.

VARIATION
Ginger Tea

For an easy antinausea tea, peel and roughly slice a ¾-inch (2-cm) piece of gingerroot into a cup, and fill with boiling water. Add 1 tsp of honey to sweeten, if preferred, and a slice of lemon. Leave to infuse for a few minutes, then drink.

Brownish-black chaste berries (***Vitex agnus-castus***) contain remarkable hormone-regulating substances, which have been shown to be effective in alleviating symptoms of premenstrual syndrome (PMS). This recipe for chaste berry vinegar can help minimize PMS-related symptoms, such as backache, stomach cramps, breast tenderness, irritability, and mood swings.

PMS

Chaste Berry Vinegar

¾ cup (200 ml) good-quality cider vinegar
½ cup (50 g) chaste berries, fresh or dried

Pour the vinegar over the berries in a jar. Seal. Shake every day for 2 weeks. Strain, and return to the jar.

USE Take 1 tsp every day.
CAUTION: Do not use if you are pregnant.

STORAGE Keeps for 6 months in a dark place.

Snack on this chewy dried-fruit treat regularly to help prevent cystitis. It is equally effective if you're suffering an acute attack. Cranberry works by preventing bacteria from attaching to the wall of the bladder, where they start multiplying.

CYSTITIS
Cranberry Fruit Leather

5 cups (500 g) fresh, ripe cranberries
superfine sugar, to taste

1 Rinse and dry the cranberries. Crush with a rolling pin to make a mash, collecting all the juice you can. Alternatively, if you prefer a smoother texture, purée in a blender.

2 Line a cookie sheet with parchment paper. Press the berry mash into the tray. Smooth the top. Place in the oven at the lowest setting (about 125ºF (50ºC), and leave for up to 12 hours. Check often to make sure the fruit does not overdry—you want a texture that holds its shape when pulled away from the parchment but does not crack or crumble.

3 Then sprinkle with sugar—as little as possible but enough to make the fruit leather palatable. Leave the sugared leather in its tray to dry out for another 12 hours, or until it is completely dry.

4 Warm the leather in a very low oven for 10 minutes, then roll it and cut into slices. Store in an airtight container on wax paper.

USE Chew on a strip as often as you like.

STORAGE Keeps in the refrigerator for about 1 month.

UNDER THE WEATHER

Echinacea lessens the severity and duration of colds and flu. Keep these ice Popsicles in the freezer to suck on when you feel the first signs of infection coming on.

COLDS AND FLU
Echinacea Popsicles

To make the tincture:
20 g fresh echinacea root
⅓ cup (80 ml) vodka

For the Popsicles:
2 medium red chilies
1½ tsp (8 cm) gingerroot
1 cup (240 ml) honey
1 packet gelatin
3¼ cups (800 ml) cranberry juice
juice of 2 large lemons

Echinacea Tincture (see above)

1 Wash and chop the echinacea root, then put in a jar and add the vodka, covering echinacea completely. Leave for 2 to 4 weeks.

2 Wash and slice the chilies. Peel and thinly slice the ginger.

3 Combine the chilies, ginger, honey, gelatin, and cranberry juice in a large saucepan, then stir and simmer for 5 minutes. Remove from heat and set aside to cool. Place a sieve over a large bowl, and pour in the hot mixture.

4 When the drained liquid is cool, stir in the lemon juice and "Echinacea Tincture." Pour into Popsicle molds or freezer trays and freeze.

USE Good when fighting cold or infection. NOTE: Contains alcohol.

STORAGE The Popsicles will keep in the freezer for 3 months.

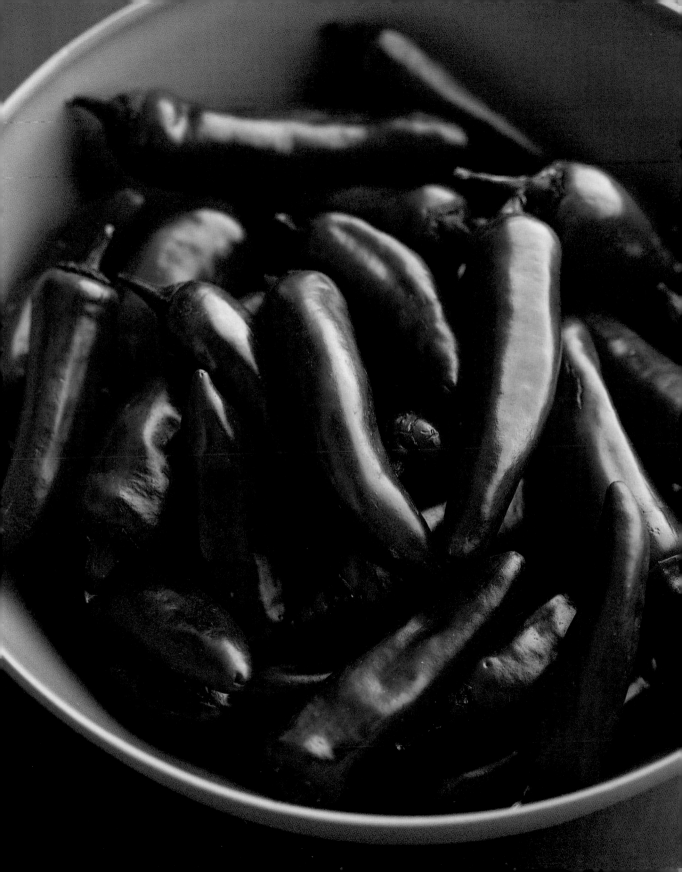

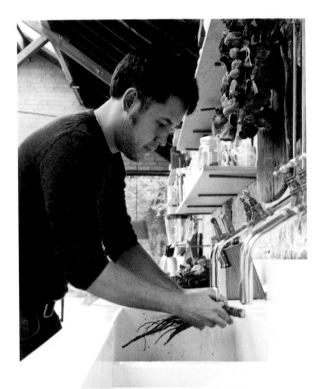
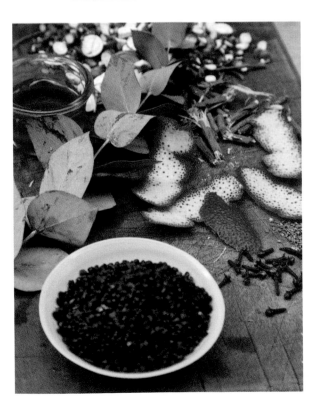
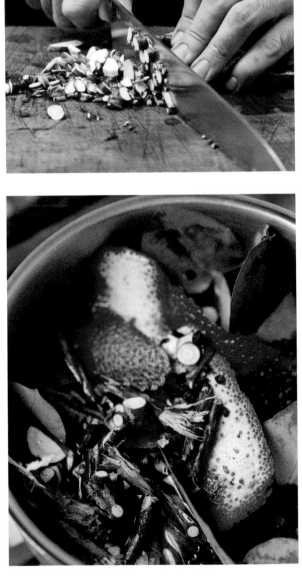

Licorice has been used for centuries as an expectorant to loosen phlegm. When mixed with marshmallow, which contains a soothing mucilage, it reduces coughing and helps to soothe sore throats. This syrup is especially good for dry or tickly coughs. Quantities differ depending on whether you use fresh or dried marshmallow root.

COUGHS AND SORE THROATS
Marshmallow and Licorice Cough Syrup

If using dried marshmallow root:
4 tbsp dried marshmallow root, coarsely chopped
2 dried licorice roots, broken into small pieces
3 heads/bunches fresh elderberries
1 tsp ground cloves
peel of 1 tangerine orange
1 tsp anise seeds
1 sprig of fresh eucalyptus leaves (about 8)
2 cups (500 ml) water
½ cup (100 ml) honey
juice of 1 lime
5 tbsp glycerin

If using fresh marshmallow root:
8 tbsp fresh marshmallow root, coarsely chopped
4 dried licorice roots, broken into small pieces
other ingredients as above

1 Put the marshmallow, licorice, elderberries, cloves, tangerine peel, anise, and eucalyptus leaves into a pan with the water. Simmer until the liquid is reduced by one-fifth. Remove the licorice and eucalyptus leaves and discard.

2 Blend the mixture in a blender until smooth. Pour back into the pan and add the honey, lime juice, and glycerin, then stir and simmer for 2 minutes.

3 Pour into sterilized, clear ½-pint (250-ml) bottles.

USE Take 2 tbsp 3 times a day.

STORAGE Keep refrigerated; use within 2 weeks.

Small red hawthorn berries (*Crataegus laevigata*), which are prolific in the fall, have been shown in clinical studies to lower blood pressure, improve coronary blood flow, and reduce the absorption of cholesterol in the body. Combined with artichokes (*Cynara scolymus*), which also contain cholesterol-lowering substances, this chewy fruit leather may help boost heart health, especially in those with borderline high levels of cholesterol. This makes a large batch—take a few pieces with you to munch on every day.

CHOLESTEROL REDUCER
Hawthorn and Artichoke Fruit Leather

4 artichokes
1 qt (1 L) water
approx. 5 cups (475 g) hawthorn berries (if using dried hawthorn berries, first cover them with water for 24 hours to rehydrate them)
1 cup (225 g) sugar
1 cinnamon stick
juice of 1 lime

1 Wash artichokes and trim the end of the stem. Then chop and place in a saucepan, cover with the water, and boil for 10 minutes, or until cooked. Remove from heat, then let to steep for 20 minutes. Strain into a bowl.

2 Preheat the oven to 200°F (100°C).

3 Place the artichoke infusion, hawthorn berries, sugar, and cinnamon stick in a pan, 20 minutes, or until the mixture is soft. Take out the cinnamon stick and mix in a blender with the lime juice. Then pour into greased baking pans, to a thickness of approximately ⅓ inch (1 cm).

4 Dry in the heated oven for 2 or 3 hours. (Check after 2 hours; leather should be chewy, but not too tough.) Let cool, then slice into bite-sized pieces.

USE Chew on a piece of fruit leather whenever you like.
CAUTION: If high blood cholesterol is suspected, you must see a doctor. This recipe may be used in addition to, not as a substitute for, proper medical treatment.

STORAGE Keep in wax paper in an airtight container in the refrigerator for up to 1 month.

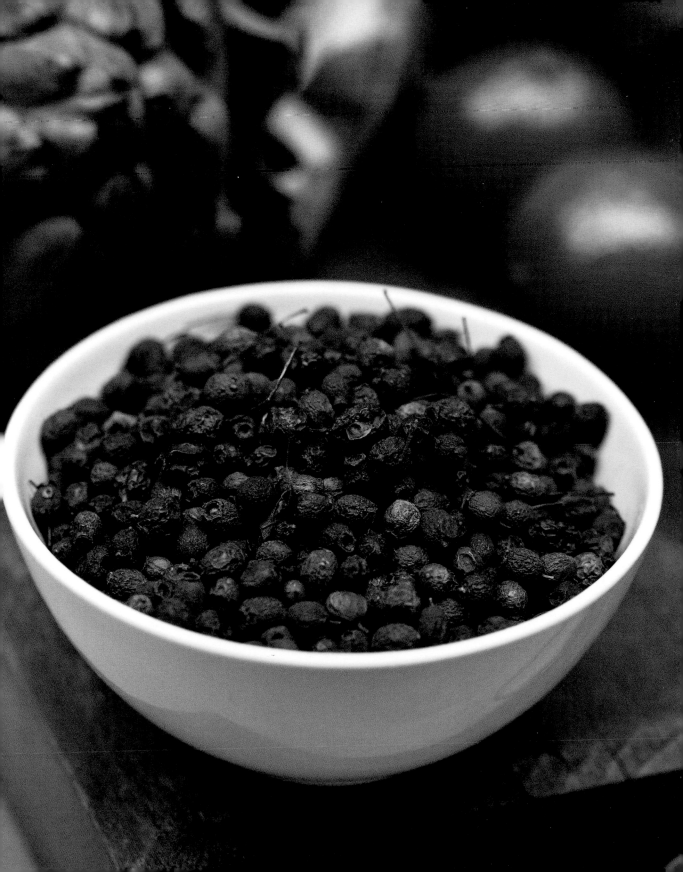

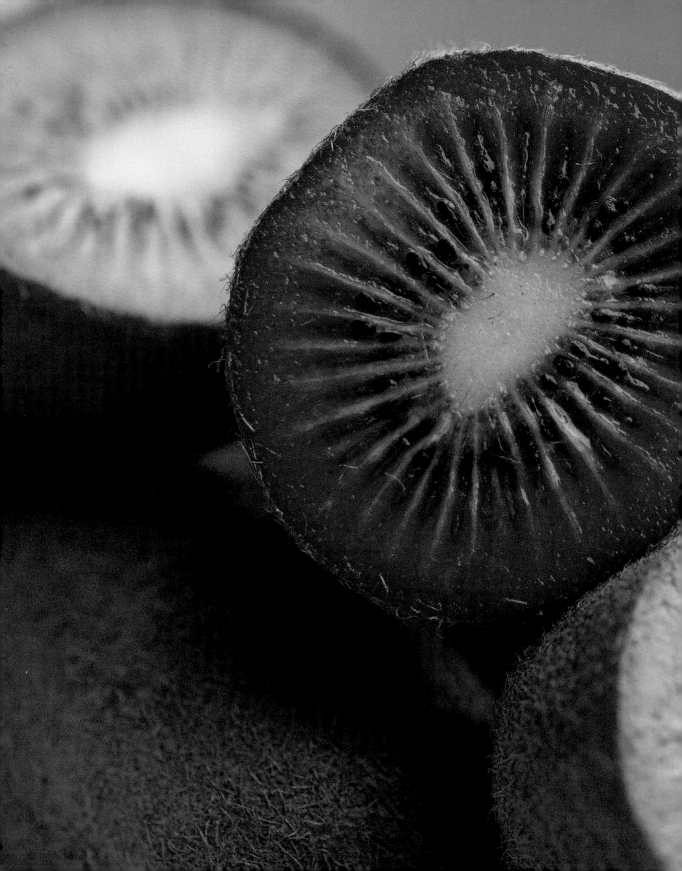

Kiwifruit, which are high in vitamin C, and feverfew (*Tanacetum parthenium*), a gentle analgesic for headaches, come together in this morning-after smoothie. The honey and kiwifruit also contain fructose, a natural sugar that has been shown to alleviate hangovers.

HANGOVER
Kiwi Morning-After Smoothie

2 cups (500 ml) freshly boiled water
3 tbsp feverfew flowers (see Resources on page 218)
3 kiwifruit, peeled
3 tbsp honey
½ tsp salt

1 Pour the water over the feverfew flowers and let steep for up to 8 minutes.

2 Place the infusion in a blender with the remaining ingredients and mix until smooth. Add more honey, if needed—feverfew flowers can be bitter. Serve at once.

STORAGE Can be stored in the refrigerator for up to 24 hours.

Lemon balm can be effective in reducing the duration and frequency of cold sores. This balm is easy to carry in a handbag or pocket and also helps to keep lips from chapping.

COLD SORES
Lemon Balm Lip Salve

21 tbsp (approx. 50 g) fresh lemon balm leaves
3 tbsp wheat germ oil
½ cup (115 ml) olive oil
1 tbsp honey
1 tbsp beeswax
5 drops tea tree essential oil

1 Finely chop lemon balm leaves. In a pan over low heat, stir and crush one third of the lemon balm leaves with the wheat germ and olive oil for 10 minutes, or until mixture starts to bubble. Remove from heat.

2 Strain the oil through a cheesecloth-lined sieve or colander into a bowl, squeezing the leaves to get out all remaining juice. Discard the squeezed leaves.

3 Repeat this process twice more with the remaining 2 batches of lemon balm leaves, using the same oil.

4 Place the oil back in the pan over low heat and add the honey and beeswax. Stir until melted, then remove from heat and stir in the tea tree oil.

5 Pour the salve into small sterilized jars, where it will set solid within 10 minutes.

USE Apply to lips whenever needed.

STORAGE Keeps for up to 1 year.

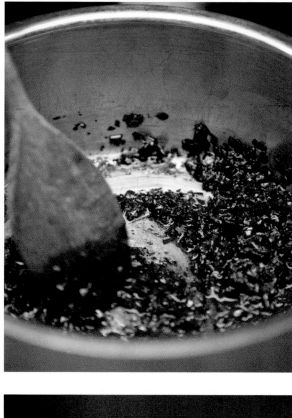
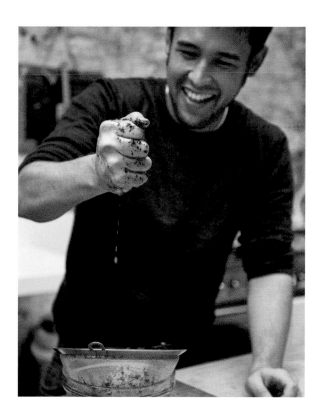
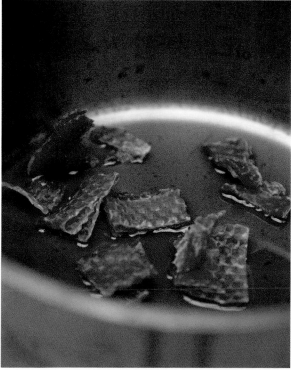
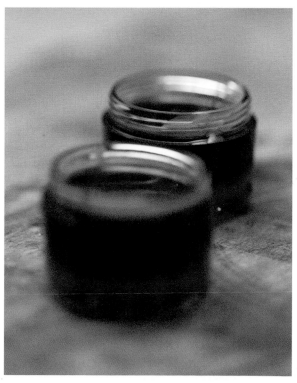

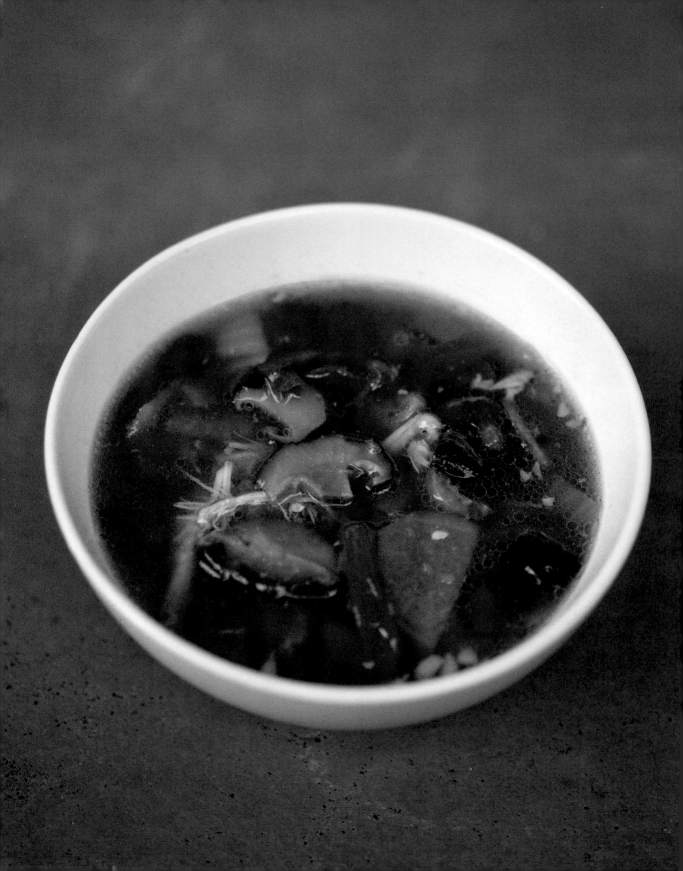

In China, soup instead of tea is the traditional way of administering health-giving herbs. This soup is packed with nutrients that help to boost immunity and generally ease the symptoms of colds and flu. Eat this soup as soon as you feel a cold coming on.

IMMUNE SYSTEM BOOSTER
Goji Berry and Shiitake Mushroom Soup

2 tbsp dried echinacea root
¾ cup (200 ml) freshly boiled water
5 tbsp goji berries, fresh or dried (see Resources on page 218)
2 qt (2 L) chicken stock (homemade or canned)
3 chicken thighs or drumsticks (preferably organic)
2 large onions, sliced
12 shiitake mushrooms, thinly sliced
2 tsp (10 cm) gingerroot, peeled and shredded
2 medium chilies, finely sliced
8 garlic cloves, chopped
extra sliced ginger and chilies, for garnish

1 Combine the dried echinacea root with the water in a bowl to make a simple infusion. In another bowl, pour just enough cold water over the goji berries to cover, and leave to rehydrate. Set the echinacea and goji berries aside and let stand.

2 Place the stock and chicken pieces in a large pan or slow cooker. Add the sliced onions, mushrooms, ginger, and chilies and place around the chicken in the pan. On a very low heat, simmer gently for 1½–2 hours, or until the chicken is tender and falls apart. Remove from heat.

3 Five minutes before serving, add the goji berries and chopped garlic. Finally, strain the echinacea infusion and add this to the soup, reheating if necessary.

4 Serve by ladling into bowls and garnishing with sliced ginger and chilies for an extra kick.

USE Makes enough for 4; serve with noodles, if desired.

Honey is the magic ingredient in this soothing syrup,
but the cherries and lemon add a zingy punch of vitamin C.

COUGHS

Cherry Cough Syrup

approx. 3¾ cups (500 g) cherries (leave the pits in)
1 lemon, sliced
1 cup (250 ml) honey

Place all ingredients in a pan with enough water to cover and simmer gently for about 30 minutes, or until the cherries are soft. Remove from the heat and strain out the solids, then allow to cool. Pour into a sterilized bottle.

USE Take 2 tbsp, as required, to soothe coughing.

STORAGE Keeps for several days in the refrigerator.

Ulcers inside the mouth often come in clusters, making eating, drinking, and even talking uncomfortable. Myrrh contains a painkilling resin that forms a film over the ulcers, while the peppermint and cloves work as an antiseptic and offer cooling relief. Used regularly for a couple of days, this mouthwash will improve symptoms and reduce discomfort.

MOUTH ULCERS
Myrrh Mouthwash

20 drops peppermint essential oil
5 drops clove oil
¼ cup (60 ml) witch hazel
1 tsp tincture of myrrh (available at your local health food store)
½ cup (120 ml) glycerin
1 cup (250 ml) cooled boiled or distilled water

Place all of the ingredients in a bowl and stir well. Filter into a large sterilized bottle.

USE Dilute with warm water (1 part in 4) and use every hour as a mouthwash or gargle to relieve pain until the soreness has disappeared. Do not swallow in large amounts.

STORAGE Keeps for 1 month.

This is a good spring soup: The nettles (*Urtica dioica*) are packed with nourishing vitamins and minerals that can help build natural immunity and protect from infections after a long winter.

RESTORATIVE
Nettle Soup

2 tbsp (25 g) butter
1 medium onion, finely chopped
2 garlic cloves, crushed
3 medium (400 g) potatoes, peeled and chopped
450 g freshly picked nettle tops (wear gloves to collect), washed
1 qt (1 L) vegetable stock
⅔ cup (150 ml) heavy cream
freshly grated nutmeg
salt and freshly ground black pepper

1 In a large pan, melt the butter and gently sauté the onion and garlic for 10 minutes. Add the potatoes and nettles and sauté for 2 minutes. Add the stock and cover, then bring to a boil and simmer for 15 minutes. remove from heat and cool.

2 Puree the ingredients with a handheld bender, then stir in the cream and season with a little nutmeg, salt, and pepper. Reheat and serve at once.

USE Makes enough for 6.

VARIATION
Nettle Pesto

This is another simple, tasty way to get the benefits of *Urtica dioica*. The young spring tips are the most tender and tastiest. Just cook a big handful of the young nettle tips (about 150 g) in boiling water for about 2 minutes. Drain, then place in a blender along with some freshly grated Parmesan, 2 chopped garlic cloves, a handful of pine nuts and about ⅓ cup (80 ml) olive oil. Blend until smooth, then spoon over freshly cooked pasta.

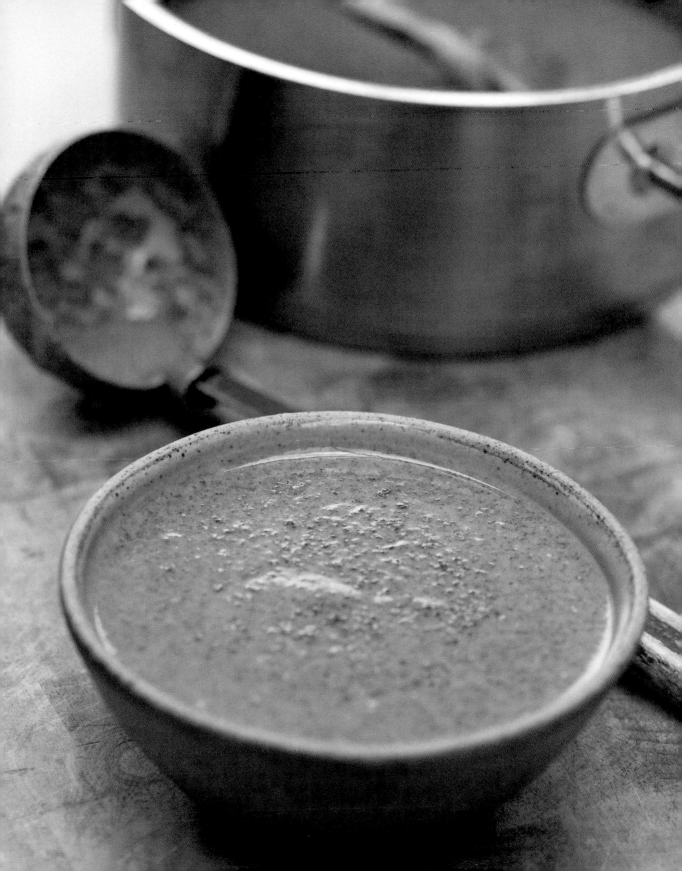

Echinacea has been shown to have a beneficial effect on the immune system, as well as a numbing effect on the throat. Add in the antiseptic properties of the cloves and sage and the cooling effect of the peppermint, and you'll get instant relief every time you use this spray.

SORE THROAT
Echinacea Throat Spray

3 cloves
5 peppermint leaves, finely chopped
5 sage leaves, finely chopped
2 tbsp (30 ml) *Echinacea purpurea* tincture
    (from natural food stores)

1 Place the cloves, peppermint, and sage leaves in a small glass bowl, then add the echinacea tincture. Cover and let stand for 2 weeks in a cool, dark place. You will see the color change gradually.

2 Strain the liquid through cheesecloth placed in a strainer, squeezing all of the liquid from the herbs by hand. Filter the liquid into a sterilized spray bottle.

USE Spray as often as needed.

STORAGE Keeps in the refrigerator for up to 1 year.

Pungent sage leaves (*Salvia officinalis*) contain antiseptic, anti-inflammatory and decongestant properties; in fact, so all-around helpful is this herb that it takes its name from the Latin verb "to save." Combined with the antibacterial and healing properties of honey, this makes a great throat soother.

SORE THROAT
Sage Honey

1 large bunch of fresh sage leaves
enough honey (buy sage honey if you can),
    to cover the leaves

1 Wash and dry the sage leaves and place in a small pan with enough honey to cover. Simmer gently for 1 hour. Allow to cool to a temperature you can handle. (Be careful: Sugar solutions and honey can become very hot and cause scalding.)

2 Strain the honey into a sterilized jar containing a sprig of sage, if desired.

USE Take 1 tsp whenever needed to soothe a sore throat. You can also use to sweeten and medicate hot lemon drinks for colds and flu; take 3 or 4 times a day when needed.

STORAGE Keeps for about 6 months.

MIND

Ginkgo is used by many people to help improve concentration, short-term memory, and reaction time. Recently there has been an enormous amount of research into the efficacy of this herb, and many of its properties are now being studied. These clinical trials have shown ginkgo to be ineffective in treating dementia or preventing Alzheimer's disease.

MEMORY ENHANCER
Ginkgo Tea

5 fresh ginkgo leaves or 2 tsp dried
1 drinking cup freshly boiled water

Add the ginkgo to the cup of freshly boiled water and let steep for 10 minutes. Strain and drink immediately.

USE Drink this tea once or twice a day.

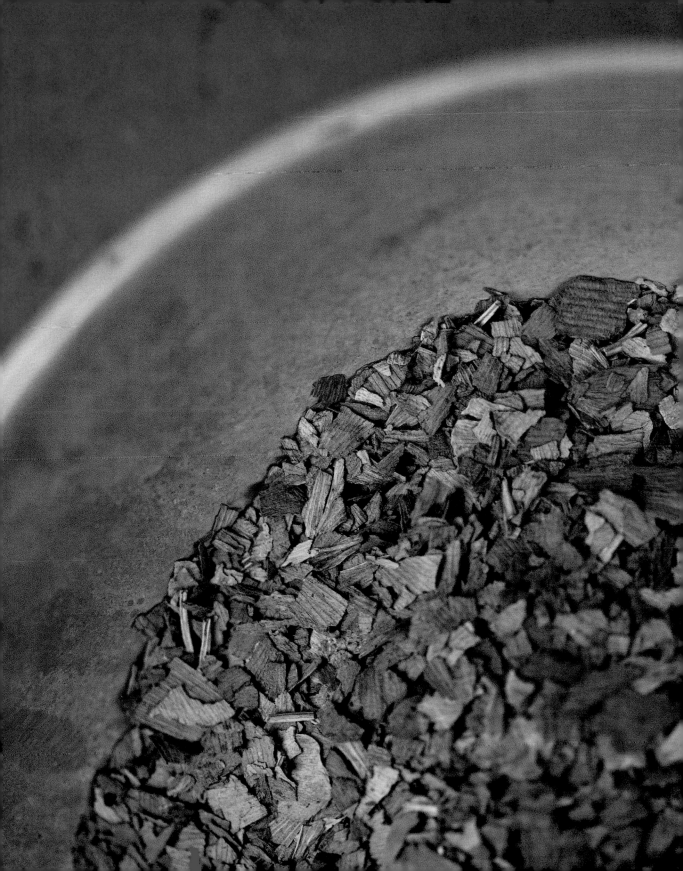

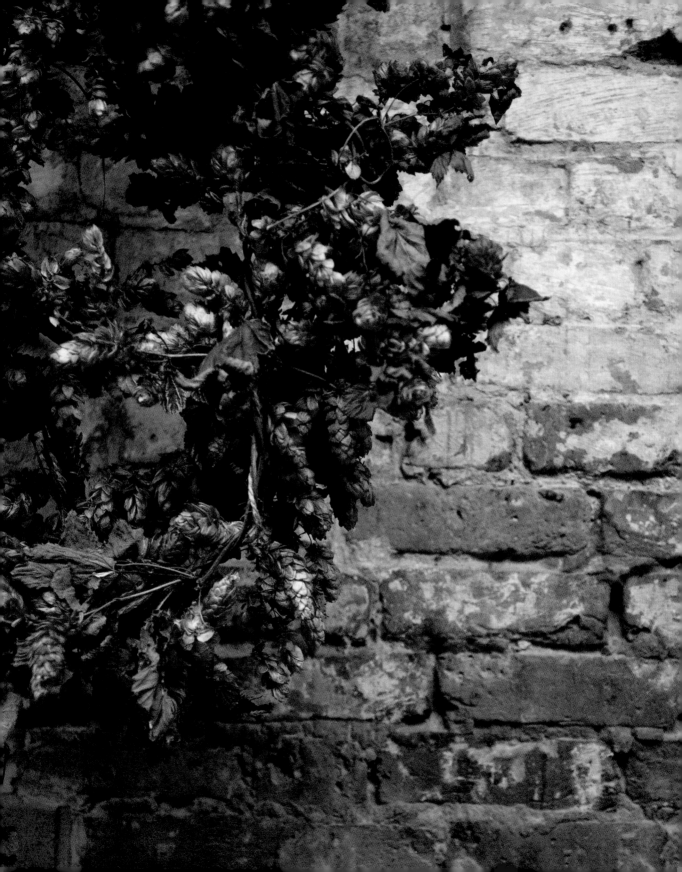

Sleeplessness—difficulty in falling asleep or staying asleep—affects 30 percent of us at some time in our lives. Hops flowers (*Humulus lupulus*) are renowned as a sleep promoter. They contain bitter acids and volatile oils that work together to soothe the nerves and promote relaxation, providing a better night's sleep without the aftereffects of prescription sleeping medications. Dry your own fresh hops if possible (see step 1 below), to retain more of the volatile oils than are normally present in store-bought preparations.

INSOMNIA
Hops Pillow for Insomnia

4 handfuls of dried hops flowers
4 handfuls of dried lavender flowers
1 standard cotton pillowcase

1 To dry your own hops and lavender, tie them in bunches and hang upside down in a well-ventilated space out of direct sunlight for 2 weeks. Alternatively, place in a low oven (about 200°F [100°C]) for 30 minutes or so until dry and crispy. Strip the flowers off the larger or harder stalks.

2 Put equal handfuls of dried hops and lavender flowers into the pillowcase, and seal the end.

USE Place the pillow under or beside your head to induce sleep.

VARIATION
Chamomile and Hops Bath

1 To make a small cheesecloth bag, place together two small squares of cheesecloth and sew together three sides. Put 1 handful (approx. 20 g) of chamomile flowers and 1 handful (approx. 20 g) of hops into the bag, then sew up the opening. Alternatively, use a clean cotton sock or cut the foot off a pair of tights, and tie the top.

2 Put the bag into the bath while the water is running, swishing it around the bath and squeezing it occasionally. The hot bathwater allows the relaxing oils in these herbs to vaporize and be inhaled.

3 Relax in the bath for at least 15 to 20 minutes.

Feverfew (*Tanacetum parthenium*), also known as bachelor's button, was mentioned in **The British Herbal** in 1772, where Sir John Hill extolled its virtues for use with "raging" headaches. Clinical studies have since shown that the fresh leaves may be effective at preventing migraines, if taken regularly. You can grow the plant in your garden.

Because the leaves taste bitter and unpleasant, it's best to add them to other food to disguise the flavor. Feverfew has also been used to treat arthritic pain.

MIGRAINE PREVENTION
Feverfew Sandwiches

2 fresh feverfew leaves
sandwich, containing filling of your choice

To aid digestion, add two fresh leaves (1 g) to a lunchtime sandwich.

Here is a simple, soothing drink to calm anxiety and promote sleep at the end of a stressful day. If you don't have valerian or lemon balm, don't worry—you can still enjoy sipping the hot drink.

ANXIETY
Valerian Hot Chocolate

Makes 3 cups
3 tbsp fresh valerian root
3 tbsp fresh lemon balm leaves
3 tsp fresh lavender flowers
6 leaves and 3 heads from fresh passionflowers
peel of 1½ oranges
3¾ cups (900 ml) whole milk
50 g dark chocolate (minimum 50% cocoa solids)
dash of vanilla extract

1 Chop the top and bottom from the fresh valerian root. Add the valerian, lemon balm, lavender, passionflowers, orange peel, and milk to a pan and gently heat for 5 to 10 minutes. Do not let mixture come to a boil. Strain.

2 Pour the infused milk back into the pan, then add the dark chocolate and vanilla extract and stir until melted. Drink at once.

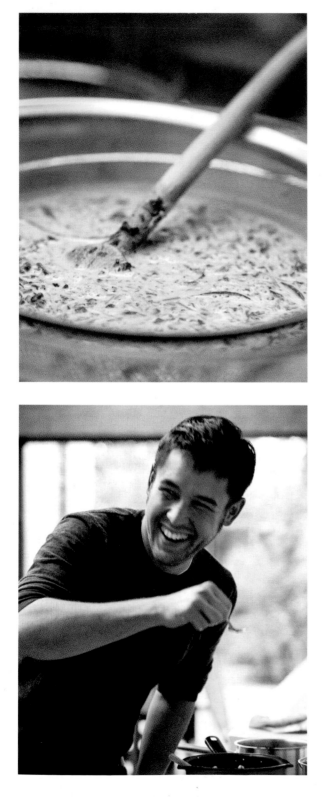
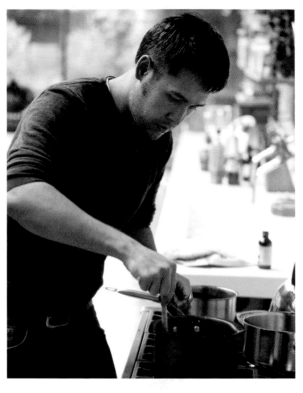
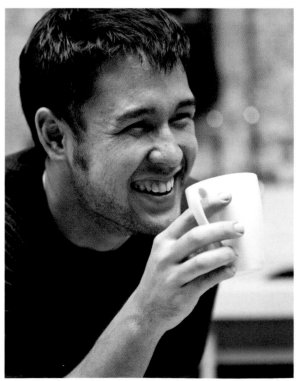

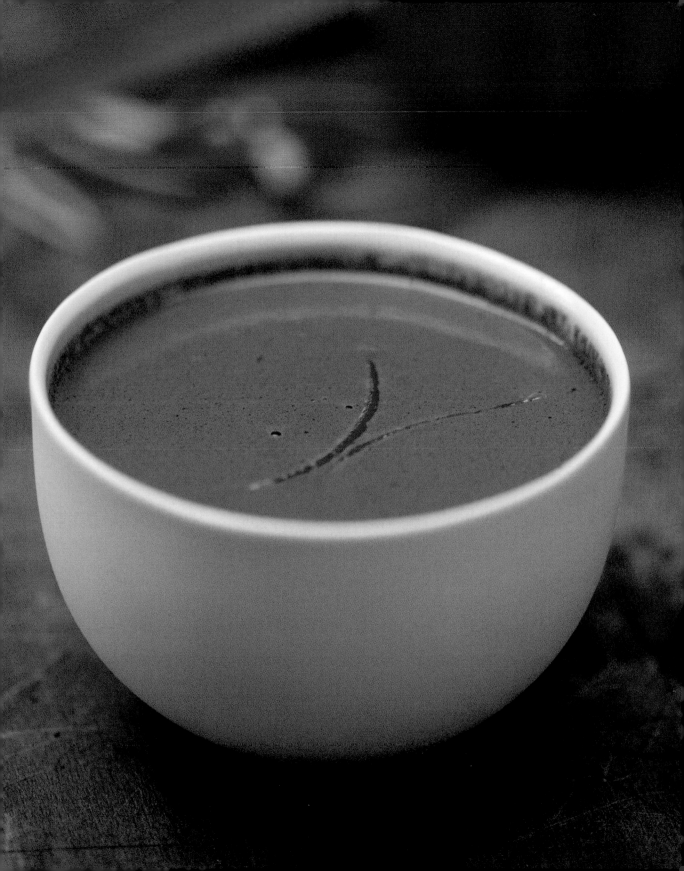

Rosemary is called the "herb of remembrance" and has traditionally been used to improve memory. For this memory-boosting tonic it's best to use southern French or California wine (for the high alcohol content).

MEMORY BOOSTER
Rosemary Wine

1 bottle of good-quality (preferably organic) wine
5 sprigs of fresh rosemary

Bruise the rosemary and place in the bottle of wine. Recork and shake every day for 2 weeks.

USE Drink one small glass daily after dinner.

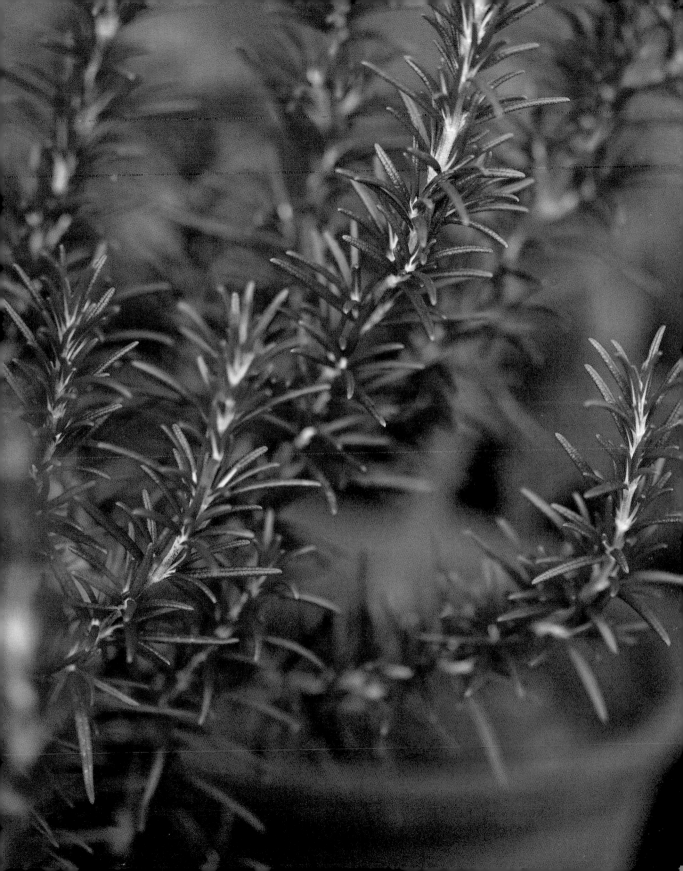

FACE AND BODY

An easy-to-make hair tonic that can be used as a final rinse after shampooing, or as a hair enhancer to stimulate growth. Either way, you'll be left with smooth, soft hair.

HAIR STRENGTHENER
Nettle Hair Tonic

1 large bunch of nettle leaves, fresh or dried
2 cups (500 ml) water
2 cups (500 ml) white wine vinegar
1 tbsp aromatic herbs
   (rosemary and lavender, for example) or 10 drops of essential oil

Place nettles, water, and vinegar in a large pot and simmer for 2 hours. Then stir in the aromatic herbs or essential oil and allow the mixture to cool. Strain through a sieve lined with cheesecloth. Filter into bottles.

USE Apply to the scalp every other night as a hair-strenthening tonic, or use as a final hair rinse after shampooing.

STORAGE Keeps for at least 1 month.

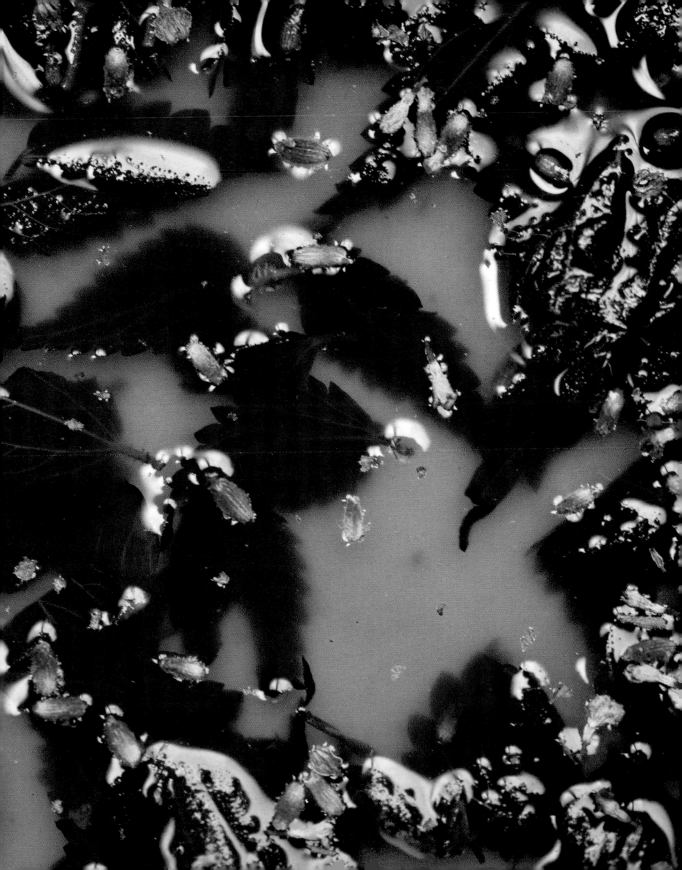

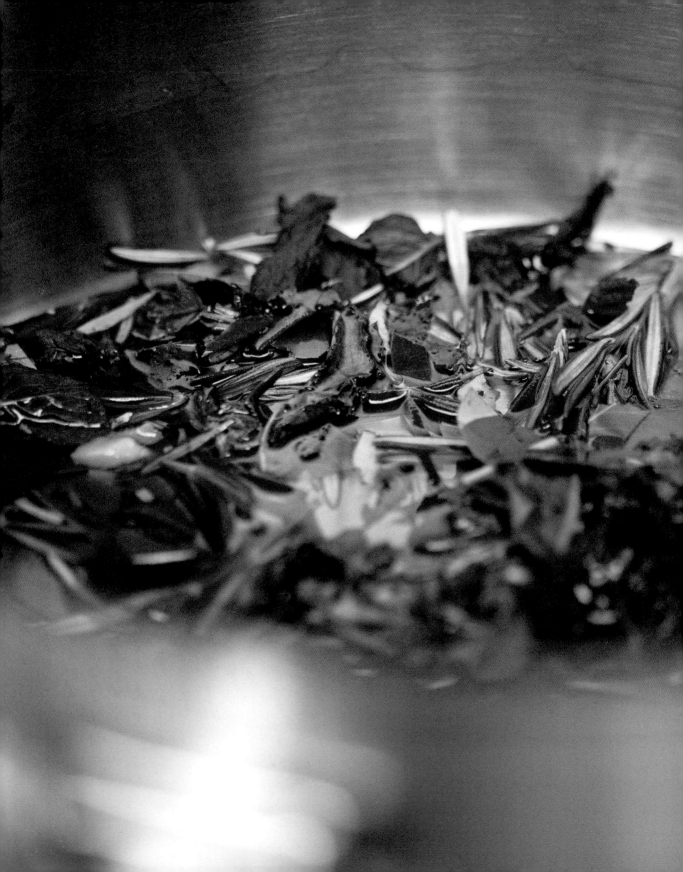

Combine the words "cosmetic" and "pharmaceutical" and you get "cosmeceutical," the name now applied to cosmetics that are supposed to have a biological effect on the body. In the West, cosmeceuticals are a new and trendy concept, but in most other traditions, medicine and cosmetics have long been viewed together—a patient is as likely to visit a shaman for limp, dull-looking hair as for indigestion. After all, a healthy person also looks good. This scrub might just seem cosmetic, but it may also offer a benefit to the circulatory system, making you look good from the inside out.

BODY SCRUB
Herbal Scrub

50 g fresh mint leaves, finely chopped
50 g fresh eucalyptus leaves, finely chopped
50 g fresh rosemary leaves, finely chopped
1 tbsp freshly ground black pepper
peel of 2 lemons
1¼ cups (300 ml) olive oil
1⅔ cups (400 g) sea salt (fine-grained)
4 tsp vitamin C powder
extra eucalyptus leaves and slices of lemon peel, for garnish

1 In a medium-size pan combine the chopped herbs, black pepper, and lemon peel, and then add the olive oil. Place on medium heat and stir, then leave for 2 minutes. Place the paste in a piece of cheesecloth over a sieve and squeeze out all the oil into a medium-size bowl below.

2 Mix the sea salt and vitamin C powder in a second medium-size bowl. Add most of the oil (reserving a little to seal the jar) and stir well. Place the mixture in a sterilized Mason jar and press down to pack well. Decorate the top with a few eucalyptus leaves and slices of lemon rind. Pour a layer of the remaining oil on top of the salt scrub to keep it airtight.

USE Apply to wet skin in the bath or shower, as needed. Scrub, then rinse off well with warm water.

STORAGE Keeps for 6 months, or 1 year in the refrigerator.

This oil is soothing in baths or for massage. You can also add a few drops to a bowl of boiling water for use as an inhalation aid.

BATH AND MASSAGE OIL
Pine and Eucalyptus Oil

¼ to ½ tsp pine or cedar resin
(see Resources on page 218)
20 fresh eucalyptus leaves
2 tsp cloves
2 cinnamon sticks
¾ cup (200 ml) almond oil

Place all the ingredients in a small pan and gently heat for 20 minutes until soft. Strain through a sieve lined with cheesecloth. Pour into a sterilized bottle with a stopper.

STORAGE Keeps for up to 6 months in a cool, dark place.

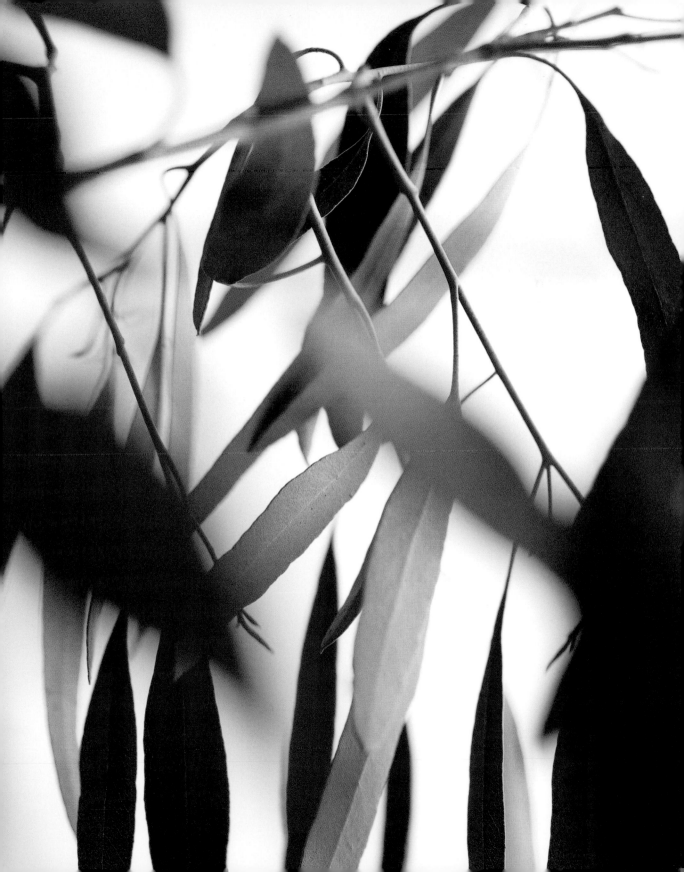

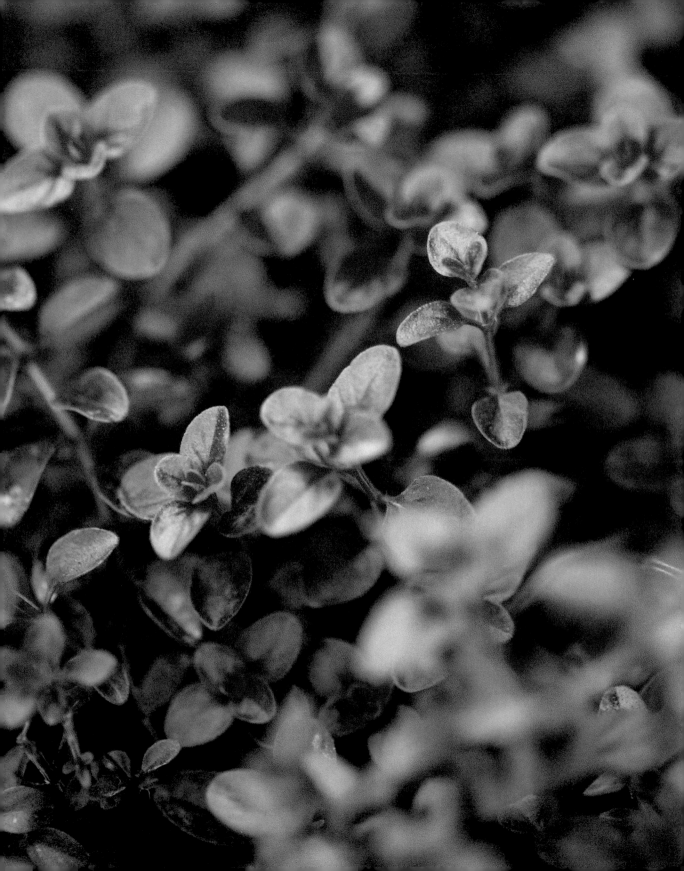

During the Middle Ages, it was thought that bad smells caused certain diseases and that sweet scents had the power to cure them. The science may be flawed, but there is some truth in the concept: Bad smells usually come from dangerous bacteria; clean-smelling substances are often antibacterial; and humans are evolutionarily hard-wired to respond to both. This natural, aluminum-free deodorant contains fragrant pine, which will help fight those odor-causing bacteria.

DEODORANT
Pine Spray

½ tsp pine resin (see Resources on page 218)
1 cup (250 ml) vodka (or just enough to cover the ingredients)
rind of 2 lemons, finely chopped
rind of 2 oranges, finely chopped
10 fresh bay leaves, finely chopped
3 tbsp fresh pine needles, finely chopped
3 tbsp fresh thyme leaves
2 tbsp glycerin
½ cup (100 ml) orange blossom water

1 With a mortar and pestle crush the pine resin until you have a very fine powder. Add 1 tbsp of vodka and stir to dissolve; the mixture should form a thin paste. Add the chopped lemon and orange rinds to the mortar and stir with a spoon to remove the last traces of sticky resin from the sides.

2 Place the resin mixture along with the bay leaves, pine needles, and thyme in a Mason jar. Add enough vodka to cover, then seal and leave in a dark place for 2 weeks to 1 month.

3 When ready, strain off the herbs using a cheesecloth-lined sieve into a jar, and stir in the glycerin and orange blossom water. Pour into a small (100 ml) glass spray bottle.

USE Do a 24-hour test on a small patch of skin before using. Shake well and apply every morning to underarms, feet, or other areas, as needed.

STORAGE Keeps for up to 1 year in a cool, dry place.

This is a gel mask that harnesses the natural fruit acids in kiwifruit, lime, and papaya to exfoliate gently, leaving the skin smooth and rejuvenated. Makes enough for 1 or 2 facial treatments.

FACE MASK
Kiwi and Papaya Face Mask

1 kiwifruit, peeled
juice of 1 lime
½ papaya
2 packets gelatin

1 Mash the kiwifruit through a sieve into a small bowl. Add the lime juice to the kiwi.

2 Scoop out the seeds from the papaya, and mash the flesh on a chopping board, using a fork (this makes it slightly easier to press through the sieve). Press the papaya through a sieve into the top of a double boiler and mix with the gelatin using a fork.

3 Put the pan with the papaya mixture over the bottom of a double boiler filled halfway with boiling water and stir constantly. As soon as mixture forms a wallpaper-paste consistency, remove from heat immediately and continue to stir. Add the kiwifruit juice slowly, bit by bit, stirring constantly. Set aside to cool.

USE When mixture is cool, apply the gel to your face, avoiding the eye area, and leave on for 10 minutes to 1 hour. Wash off with warm water.

STORAGE Most effective when used as soon as possible. Keeps in the refrigerator for up to 48 hours.

VARIATION
Lemon Jelly Peeling Face Mask

This mask uses everyday ingredients from the kitchen. Soak ½ sliced cucumber in ½ cup (125 ml) lemon juice for 30 minutes in a heat-resistant bowl. Sprinkle 1 tbsp gelatin into the juice. Place the mixture in the microwave and heat on a low setting until the gelatin dissolves completely. Set aside until cool enough to handle. Spread over the face, avoiding the eye area. Leave on for 20 minutes, then wash off with warm water.

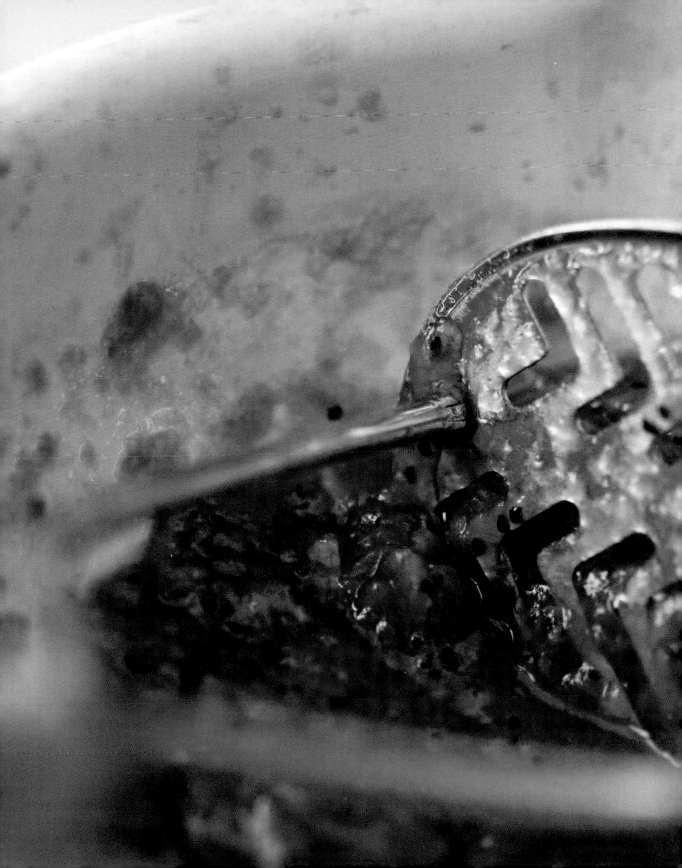

A sweet-scented and nourishing hand cream that's quick and easy to make.

HAND CARE
Rich Hand Oil

4 tsp avocado oil
2 tsp evening primrose essential oil
2 tsp vitamin E oil
5 drops sandalwood essential oil
5 drops lemon essential oil
5 drops geranium essential oil

Put all the ingredients into a small bowl and mix thoroughly. Pour into a sterilized balm jar and seal.

USE Massage a small amount into hands and feet as needed.

STORAGE Keeps for up to 6 months in a cool, dark place.

This is a flexible recipe—feel free to try different combinations of ingredients by substituting other dried flowerheads and essential oils. You'll need a large biscuit cutter to shape the bomb—ideally 1 to 1½ inches (3 to 4 cm) wide and about 1 inch (3 cm) deep. Children will love helping you make this.

BATH BOMB
Lavender Bath Bomb

5 to 6 fresh lavender sprigs
1 tbsp citric acid powder
3 tbsp baking soda
10 drops of lavender essential oil
1 tsp vegetable or almond oil

1 Preheat the oven to 350°F (180°C). Once oven has reached that temperature, turn off heat and place the lavender, hanging upside down from a rack, in the oven to dry for about 2 hours. When dry, remove the flowers from the stalks and set aside.

2 For the next stage you need to make sure that the bowl you are using, and your hands, are completely dry—otherwise the bomb will start fizzing. In a glass bowl, mix the citric acid and baking soda together. Add a few drops of lavender oil and 1 tsp dried lavender flowers, along with the vegetable or almond oil. Mix everything together with a metal spoon.

3 Place the biscuit cutter on top of a sheet of parchment paper. Put the mixture into the biscuit cutter and press down with the back of a spoon. The oil will need to evaporate so the bomb can set as a dry, hard block—let sit for a minimum of 30 minutes and preferably overnight.

STORAGE Store in aluminum foil to keep out moisture.

VARIATION
If you are making this with children, you can add ½ tsp of edible glitter into the mix to create an even more dramatic effect.

Remedies: Face and Body

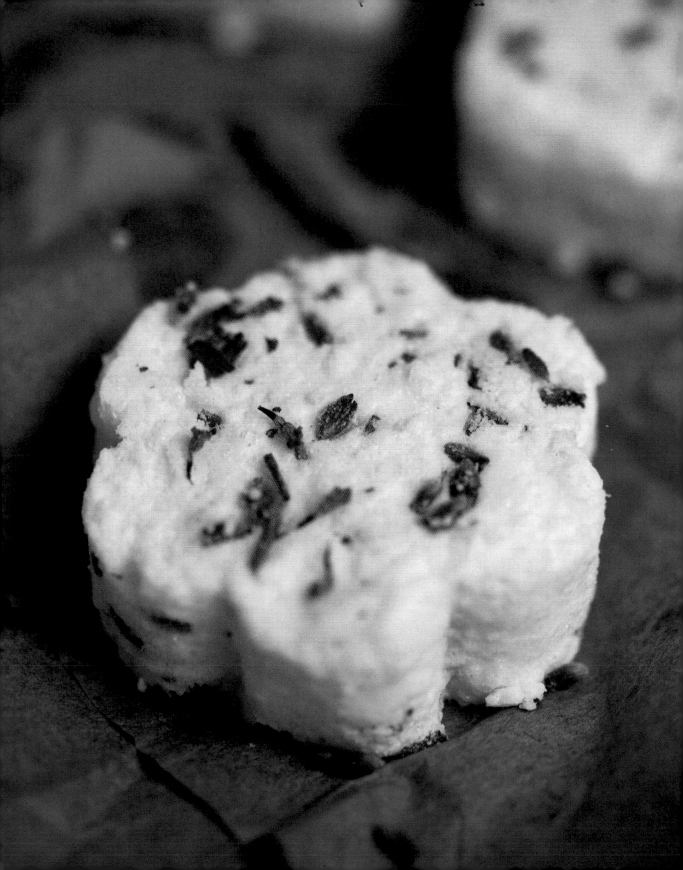

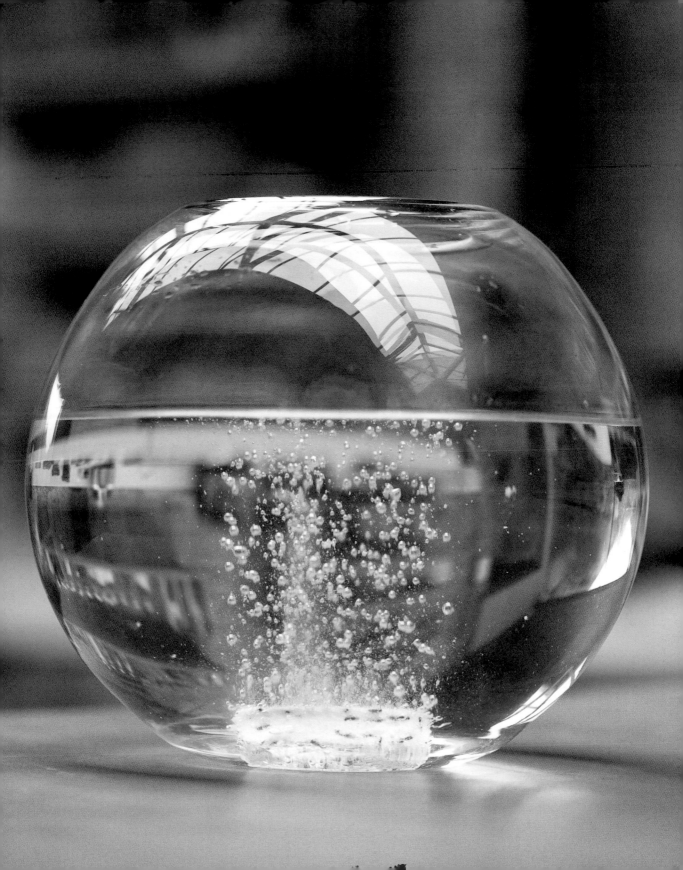

This gentle exfoliator can be used once a week. The basil oil will help to kill bacteria, and the almonds, oats and vinegar slough off dead cells to leave your skin feeling softer and looking brighter.

EXFOLIATOR
Rejuvenating Face Scrub

1 tsp ground almonds
1 tsp rolled oats
pinch of salt
½ tsp cider vinegar
2 drops of basil essential oil

Mix all of the ingredients in a small bowl. With dampened fingers roll the mixture over your face, and then rinse off.

This is a very old recipe, long touted as a panacea for both internal and external use. It makes a good toner for the face or, if made with vinegar, an effective hair rinse. Or for a more lasting version, try adding vodka to make fragrant eau de cologne.

FACE TONER/HAIR RINSE
The Queen of Hungary's Water

6 parts fresh lemon balm leaves
4 parts German chamomile (*Matricaria recutita*) flowers, fresh or dried
3 parts marigold (*Calendula officinalis*) flowers, fresh or dried
4 parts rosebuds or petals, fresh or dried
1 part sage leaves
1 part rosemary leaves, fresh or dried
1 part lemon peel
1 part fresh lovage root
apple or wine vinegar, or vodka, to cover
3 drops of lavender or rose essential oil

1 Crush all of the fresh leaves and flowers, slice the lemon peel and lovage root, and place together in a small Mason jar. Add enough vinegar or vodka to cover the plant matter, then seal the jar. Shake every day for 2 weeks.

2 Strain through a sieve lined with a double thickness of cheesecloth. Add a couple of drops of lavender or rose essential oil, then filter into small bottles.

USE Use as a facial toner, a final hair rinse, or dab on as eau de cologne (with the vodka version).

STORAGE Keeps for up to 1 year in a dark, cool place.
Note: Heat and light will destroy the fragrance.

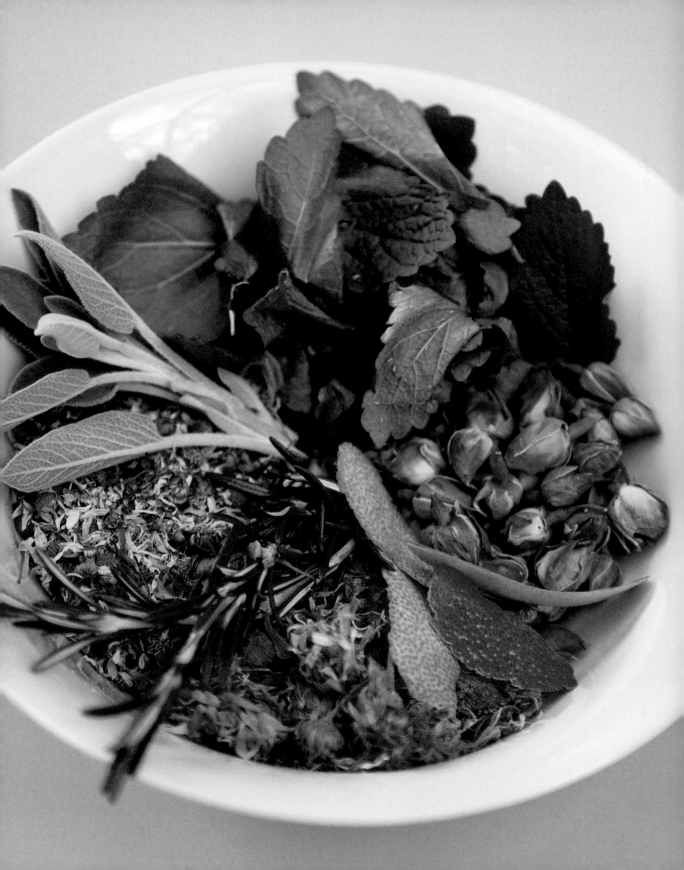

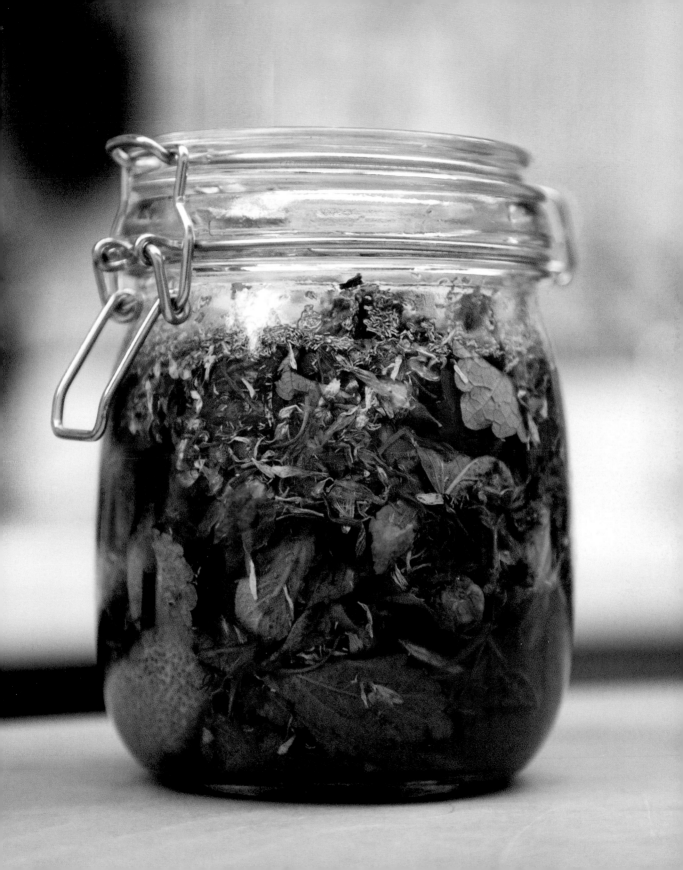

A cool, soothing gel to refresh sore or swollen eyes.

FOR SORE EYES
Cucumber Eye Gel

1 aloe vera leaf
1 small cucumber, chopped
¼ cup (50 ml) distilled extract of witch hazel (see Resources on page 218)
1 packet gelatin
1 white tea teabag
3 drops of peppermint essential oil

1 Peel and slice the aloe leaf to extract its gel. Put the cucumber and aloe gel into a blender and process until smooth. Strain the mix through a sieve to extract the juice, setting aside ½ cup (100 ml) of the strained juice.

2 Add the witch hazel to a small pan, whisk in the gelatin, and add the teabag. Gently heat the mixture until it just starts to thicken, and then remove from heat. As the mixture cools, take out the teabag, then whisk in the cucumber and aloe juice mixture and add the peppermint oil.

3 Pour the gel into a sterilized, airtight pump dispenser.

USE Apply to the eye area before bed, then wash off in the morning.

STORAGE Keeps in the refrigerator for up to 6 weeks.

This easy recipe makes a refreshing lotion to soothe tired, red eyes at the end of the day. Eyebright (*Euphrasia officinalis*) has a long history of use for eye conditions.

FOR TIRED OR RED EYES
Eyebright Eye Wash

1 tbsp dried eyebright
2½ cups (600 ml) water

Place the eyebright in a small pan and add the water. Bring to a boil and simmer for 10 minutes. Strain carefully through cheesecloth (the liquid should be clear). Set aside to cool, then pour into a glass bottle or jar.

USE Use undiluted as an eyewash 3 to 4 times a day.

STORAGE Keeps in the refrigerator for up to 1 week.

VARIATION
Chamomile and Marigold Eye Lotion

This sweet-smelling eye lotion is packed with soothing anti-inflammatory properties. Great for at the end of a heavy day in front of a computer screen.

1 Place 1 tsp each of chopped German chamomile (*Matricaria recutita*) and marigold (*Calendula officinalis*) flowers, rose petals, and fennel seeds in a glass bowl. Add 2 cups (500 ml) of hot (not boiling) water and let steep for 30 minutes.

2 Strain carefully through a double layer of cheesecloth, then filter again, to ensure lotion is very clear. Pour into a sterilized glass bottle. Use as an eyewash (diluted with a little warm water) 3 to 4 times a day. Keeps in the refrigerator for 1 week.

Are you looking for a simple, natural soap that doesn't irritate dry or sensitive skin? This soap is good for delicate and mature skins, and also looks pretty studded with rosebuds and petals. Your skin will feel softer and more nourished, too, because of the glycerin, which attracts moisture to the skin. These little soaps also make great gifts for friends and family members.

GLYCERIN SOAP
Gentle Soap

Makes about 15 small soaps
2 cups (500 ml) orange or rose flower water
2 cups (500 ml) glycerin
½ bar unperfumed white soap, grated
50 drops of rose geranium essential oil
1 handful of rose petals, chopped, or rosebuds (optional)

1 Place the flower water, glycerin and grated soap in the top of a double boiler. Place pan over bottom portion of double boiler filled halfway with boiling water. Stir mixture continuously until the soap dissolves, then remove from heat. Add the rose geranium essential oil and mix well. Drop the rose petals or buds into the mixture, if using, and stir.

2 Pour into soap molds (you can buy these online) or make a soap "loaf" by pouring mixture into a small square or rectangular straight-sided china dish, making sure the petals and buds are evenly distributed throughout. Let cool for at least 2 days. Cut the soap loaf into bars before using.

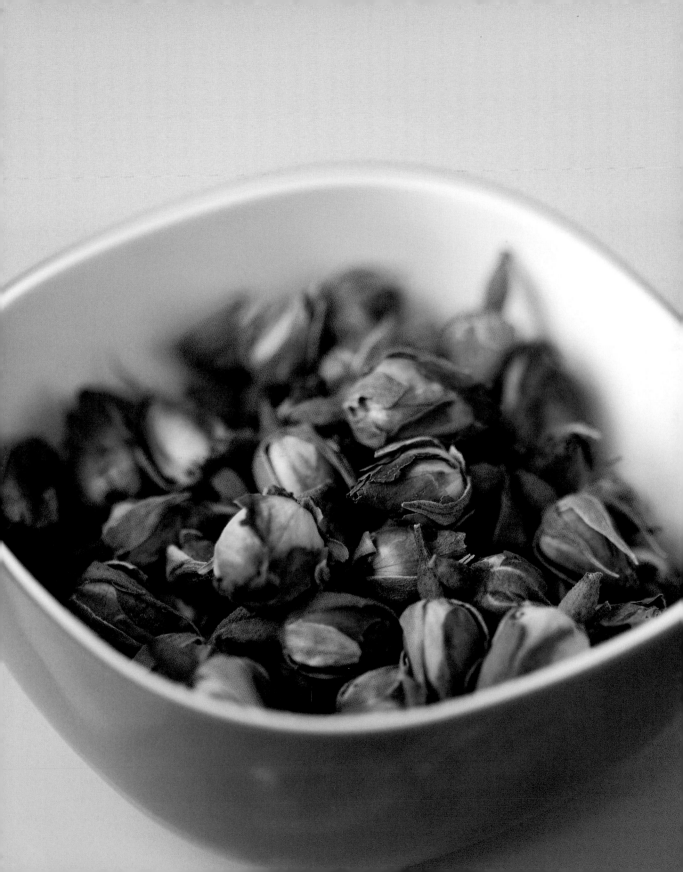

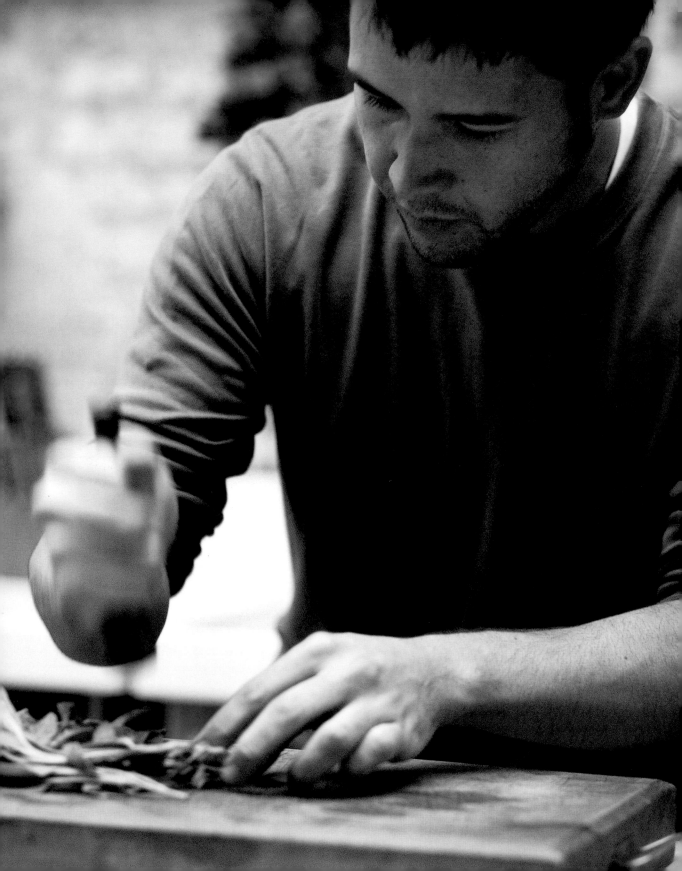

Reduce and soothe swollen gums with this germ-killing tooth powder, which has antiseptic and astringent properties. Nonabrasive, this sea salt and sage combo works to remove plaque and freshen breath without damaging enamel, so it can be used by all ages.

PLAQUE REMOVER AND GUM SOOTHER
Sage and Sea-Salt Tooth Powder

1 cup (350 g) sea salt
100 g fresh sage leaves

1 Pound the salt and sage leaves, until the leaves are well coated with salt.

2 Spread the mixture on a cookie sheet and place in the oven. Set temperature at the lowest setting and bake about 20 minutes until mixture dries completely. Check occasionally because the length of time required for drying will depend on the oven temperature and on the salt.

3 Using a coffee or salt grinder, grind mixture to a fine powder (this is easy once the mixture is dry), then put in a shallow, wide-mouthed sterilized jar with a lid to keep it airtight.

USE Use as you would toothpaste, and brush teeth morning and night.

STORAGE Keeps very well if stored in an airtight container. Use until the aroma of sage has dissipated.

Lip balms are easy to make, and this one is both nourishing and gently antiseptic. It will stop lips from getting chapped and sore—or rescue them if they already are. Make sure you use scented, organically grown roses—unscented varieties may not have the necessary properties, and it's best to avoid the chemicals used on many commercially grown roses.

CHAPPED LIPS
Beeswax Lip Balm

For the herb oil:

1 large handful (approx. 20 g) rose or marigold (*Calendula officinalis*) petals (scented and organically grown)

1 cup (250 ml) almond oil

For the lip balm:

1 cup (250 ml) rose or marigold herb oil (see above)

2 to 3 tbsp beeswax

1 tsp honey

1 tsp vitamin E oil

1 tsp aloe vera gel (extracted from the center of fleshy leaves), optional

1 Soak the rose or marigold petals in the oil for at least 5 days, in full sunlight in summer or in a warm place in winter. While the liquid is slightly warm, strain through a fine-mesh sieve lined with cheesecloth, squeezing the petals to extract the oil and scent.

2 Place the oil in the top of a double boiler and place pan over bottom portion of double boiler filled halfway with boiling water. Add the beeswax while stirring continuously. When beeswax has dissolved, add the honey, vitamin E oil, and aloe vera gel, if using, stirring continuously. Pour mixture into a small, sterilized jar with a wide neck, and cap tightly. The balm will harden as it cools.

USE Apply as needed to chapped or cracked lips.

STORAGE Keeps at least 6 months, preferably in a refrigerator.

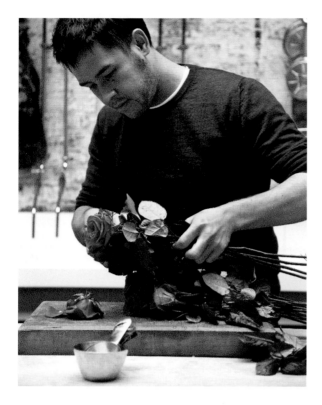

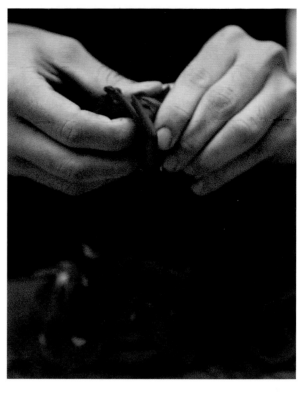

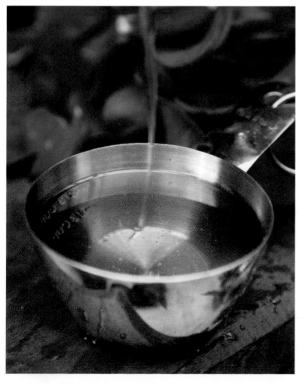

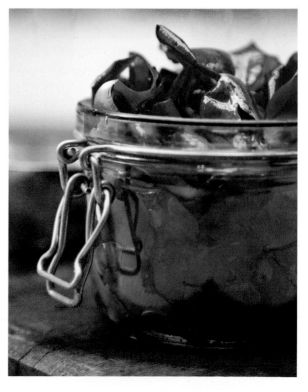

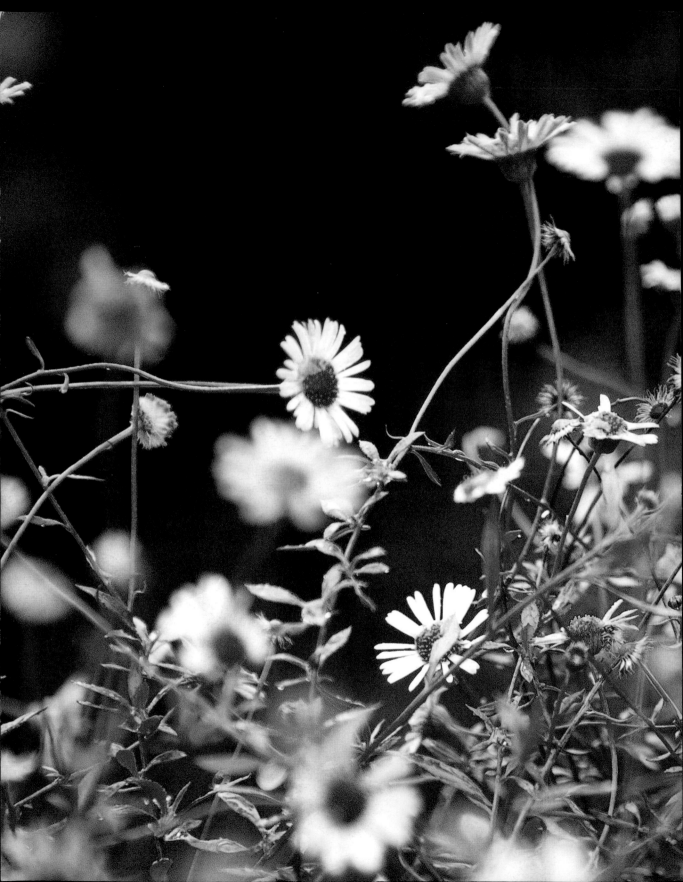

top 100 medicinal plants

The biggest challenge to those new to making herbal remedies is the sheer number of potential medicinal plants to choose from—with scientists' latest estimates clocking in at up to 50,000 species. With unpronounceable Latin names and unfamiliar growing techniques at every turn, how do you know where to start? The good news is that a huge number of the most useful species are also conveniently well known and already may be growing in your window box, popping up between the cracks of your patio, or sitting in your spice rack. Mint, thyme, and even dandelions and nettles might not seem like cutting-edge drugs, but trapped within the cells of these species are biologically active chemicals with proven medicinal properties—many of which are commonly found in over-the-counter drugs.

But perhaps the most exciting news for horticultural novices is that medicinal herbs are normally the easiest of plants to grow. In fact, many are actually invasive weeds in their country of origin—meaning that if you can grow a weedy nettle, you can grow a medicinal herb garden. You don't need a huge plot or hours of dedication, either: Herbs can be grown in any spot with water, light, and air, whether that's a sprawling country estate or a tiny window box. In fact, I've grown herbs like basil, mint, and watercress in glasses of water on a kitchen windowsill. Just pop a couple of cut stems into a glass and treat them exactly as you would a vase of flowers. They will quickly produce roots and grow happily for months on end.

To get you started, we have created an index of the top 100 medicinal plants. Or if you choose not to grow your own, look for them in your local supermarket or local garden center (see the Resources section on page 218).

FRUIT

Anise/Aniseed
Pimpinella anisum

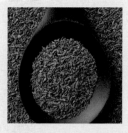

Anise is the fruit of a small annual plant grown widely in warmer parts of the world. Its licorice-like smell and sweet flavor make it popular as a cooking spice and to flavor confectionery such as anise balls and alcoholic drinks, like raki. Anise helps loosen upper-respiratory congestion and is often used in cough medicines and lozenges (see Marshmallow and Licorice Cough Syrup, page 103).

It has traditionally been used as a digestive aid, helping to soothe dyspepsia, colic, bloating, and gas, and to control nausea and vomiting. It's also reputed to increase libido—it has mild estrogenic properties and in some cultures is given to breastfeeding mothers to increase milk production. And it's a good, all-around odor-buster that masks unpleasant smells and is used to help freshen breath (see Thyme Sweet Breath Spray and Mouthwash, page 41). CAUTION: Do not use during pregnancy.

GROWS/WHERE TO FIND
> natural food stores

Bilberry
Vaccinium myrtillus

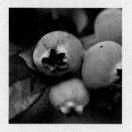

The blue–black fruits of the bilberry—or whortleberry, as it's sometimes called—is a summer delicacy that achieved mythic status after World War II, when British fighter pilots reported increased night vision after eating bilberry jam. Although that claim is unsubstantiated, trials have shown compounds in bilberries have potent antioxidant properties that contribute to the herb's many benefits, particularly for vision and eye health. It has been shown to have very positive effects on eye disorders caused by high blood pressure or diabetes. It can also help prevent cataracts and lessen glaucoma. The active ingredients are antioxidants and free-radical scavengers called anthocyanosides, which are also anti-inflammatory and anti-aging. These have been shown to help significantly with vascular problems such as varicose veins and hemorrhoids, as well as extremely painful periods and water retention. The leaves can be made into a tea (see Using Plants, page 34), which is a popular remedy for diarrhea and stomach cramps.

GROWS/WHERE TO FIND
> best in acidic soil—or it will yellow
> doesn't like being moved
> if potting, place in large pot
> does better in exposed site
> fruits best in full sun
> available in late summer

Blackcurrant
Ribes nigrum

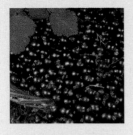

Blackcurrant oil is the richest plant source of gamma-linolenic acid (GLA). (The best source is borage oil.) It's used to treat long-lasting inflammatory skin conditions like eczema, as well as PMS, breast pain, mild hypertension, and rheumatic disorders. Blackcurrant oil outperforms evening primrose oil for rheumatoid arthritis, though it needs to be taken for six months for best effect. As the oil comes from the seeds, it's probably easier to buy rather than make at home, because you'll need very large quantities of fruit. You can, however, make the leaves into tea (see Using Plants, page 34) for use as a mild diuretic, to lower blood pressure, and alleviate sore throats and swollen glands. The berries themselves are also antiviral, protecting against flu.

Blackcurrant Gargle: Heat 2 tbsp blackcurrant leaves, chopped finely, in a pan with 1 cup (250 ml) water. Cover and simmer for 15 minutes. Strain, then cool. Use twice a day.

GROWS/WHERE TO FIND

> easy to grow
> full sun
> add lots of organic matter to soil for high nitrogen levels during growing season
> fruits on 1-year-old wood
> prune back old wood in autumn
> don't grow near pine trees, because these harbor damaging rust/fungus
> apply net to ward off birds
> buy seed oil from natural food stores

Black Mustard Seeds
Brassica nigra

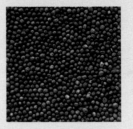

Mustard has a very hot flavor, and when applied on the body, it also works by heating. It's a counterirritant, causing reddening of the skin as blood rushes to the spot, and this increased blood flow can help reduce inflammation. Mustard plasters—a strong poultice of crushed mustard seeds and flour (see also Chili Plasters, page 91)—were traditionally applied to the chest to bring relief from chest colds, bronchial infections, and rheumatic pains. The essential compounds are found in the seeds, which are produced in black pods borne by the striking yellow flowers in late summer. Add just a few drops of seed oil to a massage-oil base and rub into stiff joints, aching muscles, and cold extremities to improve circulation. CAUTION: Mustard seed is extremely powerful and can cause skin irritation or burns. But in the right amount, you'll find it invigorating.

To make a reviving foot bath for sore feet, place 1 or 2 tbsp crushed seeds in a cheesecloth bag or cut off the foot from a pair of panty hose and tie the top. Pour 2 qt (2 L) boiling water over cheesecloth. Allow to cool a little, then soak feet for a few minutes. Rinse. (See also Hot Chili and Mustard Foot Oil, page 70.)

GROWS/WHERE TO FIND

> annual
> easy to grow from seed
> prefers light soil and sunshine
> harvest pods in late summer, tap to let the seeds out, then dry in a cool, well-ventilated space

Borage
Borago officinalis

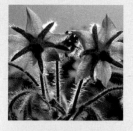

Borage grows like wildfire, its bright blue star-shaped flowers spreading seed prolifically. It has been used for centuries in inflammatory and rheumatic conditions, to treat depression, as a diuretic, and to promote sweating in fevers. Nowadays, the plant is cultivated mostly for its seeds, which are made into an oil known as starflower oil or borage seed oil. This oil is the richest plant source of gamma-linolenic acid (GLA)—greater than either evening primrose oil or blackcurrant oil. GLA is an omega-6 fatty acid used to treat dermatitis, arthritis, eczema, mastalgia, PMS, as well as the pain, tingling, and numbness caused from diabetes.

Starflower oil can also reduce joint swelling, tenderness and pain in rheumatoid arthritis, and improve the condition and function of skin, especially in the elderly. It's easy to grow borage in the garden, but it's probably not worth it for the seeds—you need to take large regular doses of the oil (1 or 2 g of GLA, or 3 to 12 capsules a day, for at least six months). Buy it at your local pharmacist instead.

CAUTION: Don't take borage leaves internally, because they contain compounds that can damage the liver. The flowers and seeds are safe, however.

GROWS/WHERE TO FIND
> drugstores and natural food stores

Caraway
Carum carvi

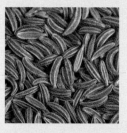

Caraway is not a common sight despite being very easy to grow in gardens or pots. Umbrella-like clusters of tiny white blooms flower from June to August, and each flower stem contains two seeds. These are dried and used in herbal remedies to soothe stomach complaints in both children and adults. Caraway helps aid digestion, ease pains, expel trapped gas, and soothe bloating (see "Four Winds" Tea, page 49). Mixed with peppermint oil, it reduces reflux and relieves heartburn.

To dry caraway seeds: In late August or when seeds are ripe, cut plants at ground level, tie stalks in small bundles, and hang upside down in a dry, well-ventilated space with sheets of wax paper below to catch the seeds.

GROWS/WHERE TO FIND
> biennial
> prefers full sun
> needs free-draining soil
> sow seeds in September directly into ground or buy fledgling pot plants from nurseries
> don't transplant because doesn't tolerate root disturbance
> self-seeds in autumn

Chaste Tree
Vitex agnus-castus

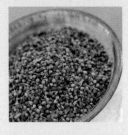

This aromatic plant is a native of the Mediterranean. Its prolific spikes of mauve flowers are followed in autumn by small, dark berries, which taste peppery and can be used fresh or dried in remedies. The berries are highly regarded as one of the best natural hormone regulators for women. They contain a range of essential compounds that seem to raise levels of the hormone progesterone during the second half of the menstrual cycle—although the exact process is not yet understood. This has significant benefits for a wide range of disorders, relieving PMS and menstrual breast pain, helping with irregular bleeding, and diminishing hormone-related acne. In one study of infertile women, chaste tree extract taken for 3 months doubled the rate of pregnancies (from 10 percent to 21 percent). It's also suggested as a remedy to relieve menopausal symptoms.

Although chaste berries stimulate the female hormone system, they seem to have the opposite effect on men. Monks used to take the berries to reduce sexual desire and help them stay "chaste," which is why they are also known as monk's pepper.

CAUTION: Don't use during pregnancy or while breastfeeding.

GROWS/WHERE TO FIND
> shrub, grows to 16 feet (5 m)
> does well in most soils
> prefers sun
> purple flowers followed by dark fruits
> you can buy standardized extracts (which have higher dosages than fresh berries) from natural food stores

Cherry
Prunus avium

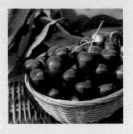

Sweet cherry trees are cultivated in gardens, and the fruit, stalks, and even the bark are used in a variety of sweet-tasting plant remedies. The fruit is packed with vitamins A, B, and C, as well as the minerals calcium and magnesium, so it makes a good general immune-system booster in cold remedies and cough syrups. Cherry also has a reputation for lowering uric-acid levels and has long been used in the treatment and prevention of gout and arthritis—though as yet there is no scientific evidence to support its use. Cherry stalks are anti-inflammatory and, when taken as a tincture or tea, can soothe dry, irritating coughs. The white inner bark can also be dried (harvest bark by pruning off small branches, stripping white inner bark and leaving to dry) and made into a cough syrup, but it will be tastier if you add some cherries for extra flavor. In large quantities, cherries are both diuretic and laxative—just don't eat too many at once.

Cherry Stalk and Apple Tea: Put 30 g cherry stems, 3 apples (cored and sliced), and 1 qt (1 L) of water into a pan. Bring to a boil and simmer for 25 minutes, or until the apples are soft. Strain. Drink as a tea 2 or 3 times a day for dry and irritating coughs.

GROWS/WHERE TO FIND
> prefers full sun
> can be fan-trained
> needs damp soil
> self-sterile, so plant two varieties to ensure pollination
> pick fruit when fully ripe (just before splitting)

Cranberry
Vaccinium macrocarpon

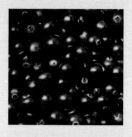

Cranberry is a sharp, sour fruit grown mostly in wet meadows in North America. Although best known as an accompaniment to Christmas dinner, it has a long history of treating cystitis and other urinary tract infections. It is thought to work by preventing bacteria from sticking to the lining of the urinary tract and increasing the acidity of urine. If you suffer recurrent bouts of cystitis, regularly eating Cranberry Fruit Leather (see page 99) or drinking homemade cranberry juice can help prevent further outbreaks (commercial juices are usually high in sugar). Cranberry is also used to help relieve the symptoms of acute attacks of cystitis, but you must check first with your family doctor to make sure it is cystitis and nothing more serious.

Cranberry and Apple Crush: Put 115 g cranberries, ¾ cup (250 ml) clear apple juice, and 1 cup water in a pan and bring to a boil. Simmer until cranberries are soft. Strain. Drink as often as necessary, adding a little sugar to taste.

GROWS/WHERE TO FIND
> best in wet acidic soil
> prefers sun or light shade
> can be grown in pots (don't allow to dry out)
> best in open ground away from strong winds

Elderberry
Sambucus nigra

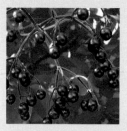

Elderflowers are often made into health-giving cordials and teas, but tiny black elderberries are less commonly used—perhaps because they have a very short season. However, the berries contain many of the same essential compounds as the flowers and are traditionally used as an anti-inflammatory to soothe coughs, sore throats, and bronchial infections and to make sinus conditions looser. Elderberry has powerful antiviral properties that combat various flu strains and have been shown to shorten the duration of flu attacks, so it is extremely useful for children and the elderly during winter months. Take as a tincture or, for children, make into a syrup (see Using Plants, page 34). CAUTION: Unripe berries may cause vomiting and diarrhea.

Elderberry Throat Gel: Fill a small Mason jar with ripe elderberries, then cover with diluted gelatin. Leave in a warm place for 2 weeks. Strain through cheesecloth, squeezing well. Pour into a sterilized bottle. Adults: Take 2 tsp 3 times a day for coughs and sore throats.

GROWS/WHERE TO FIND
> easy to grow
> vigorous—often considered a weed
> fruit ripens best in full sun
> harvest only ripe berries in September
> use a fork to strip berries from stems

Evening Primrose
Oenothera biennis

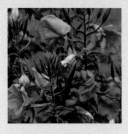

Evening primrose is a remarkable plant. During the day, it looks like any ordinary scrubland plant—in fact, it's classed as a weed in the United States, where it grows wild in open spaces and roadsides across the country. But in the evening, the yellow flowers open to welcome the moths that pollinate them overnight. Every part of the plant is edible: The nutty roots are boiled and eaten as vegetables; the leaves are eaten as greens; the seeds were traditionally dried and chewed by Native Americans.

Today the plant is cultivated mostly for its prolific seeds, cased in fluffy seed capsules, which are pressed to make evening primrose oil. Like borage, evening primrose oil is a rich source of gamma-linolenic acid (GLA), an essential fatty acid that can't be made in the body but which is essential for growth and bone health and to regulate metabolism.

Evening primrose is often recommended for the symptoms of premenstrual syndrome (sore breasts, irritability, and bloating) and menopause. It has been shown to help with the itchiness, scaling, and inflammation of eczema, to lower blood pressure slightly, and to soothe ulcerative colitis.

For best effects, you'll need to take the oil internally for 6 months or more, but the plant is still worth growing for its unusual habits and edible roots and leaves.

GROWS/WHERE TO FIND
> biennial
> thrives on neglect
> best in a low-nutrient soil
> prefers sun
> buy oil from pharmacies and natural food stores

Fennel
Foeniculum vulgare

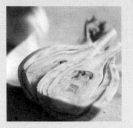

Fennel's beautiful feathery leaves and anise-flavored bulbs are used in cooking, but it's the seeds that are prized in herbal remedies. Fennel relieves bloating, flatulence, and stomach upsets of all kinds, and it was traditionally used for centuries to soothe colic. It's also recommended for menstrual pain and disorders, perhaps because of its mild estrogen-promoting qualities, and has been shown to increase breast-milk flow in nursing mothers. If you're trying to lose weight, fennel might help: It has long been used as an appetite-suppressant. Make the seeds into a tea, tincture, or oil (see Using Plants page 34) and take every day.

To dry seeds, gather flowerheads in late September/October, spread on wax paper, and leave in warm, well-ventilated space, turning every few days. Shake or comb out.

Fennel Tea for Colic: Place 1 tbsp fennel seeds in a pan with 1½ cups (400 ml) water. Simmer for 10 minutes. Strain and cool. Give 1–2 tsp when needed, not more than twice per hour.

GROWS/WHERE TO FIND
> likes a sunny spot
> dislikes wet soil
> can tolerate short drought
> attracts wildlife, including slugs and snails

Fig
Ficus carica

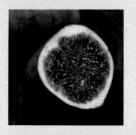

Syrup of figs has been used for hundreds of years as an effective and gentle laxative suitable for all ages. Figs work as a demulcent, soothing and protecting the bowels, and are also nutritious and very high in soluble fiber, which helps the bowels work more efficiently. Used in remedies alongside a stronger laxative such as senna (see Syrup of Figs, page 46), figs help soothe and prevent stomach pains and cramping. The roasted fruit was traditionally mashed and made into a poultice for abscesses in the mouth. Surely worth a try; at least it will taste good!

GROWS/WHERE TO FIND
> prefers slightly alkaline, free-draining soil
> place in very sunny position
> restrict roots with rocks or place in a pot to encourage fruit production
> if grown in pots, winter in frost-free conditions
> fruit usually appears one summer but doesn't ripen until the following summer
> buy fresh from natural food stores or supermarkets

Goji Berries
Lycium barbarum

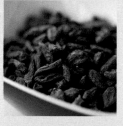

Goji berries sound exotic and are used as a superfood in Chinese medicine. In recent years, goji berries have become a fashionable cure-all. They are claimed to lower cholesterol, protect the liver, improve eyesight and dizziness, reduce the side effects of chemotherapy, boost circulation, and even improve sexual performance in men. What is certain is that the berries contain antioxidants and high levels of vitamin C, which can help various degenerative conditions and thus help improve memory and eyesight. They also contain certain sugars that are thought to enhance immune function and protect against colds and flu (try Goji Berry and Shiitake Soup, page 111). In other words, these berries are really good for you.
To make Goji Berry Tea, infuse 30 g fresh or dried berries in 2 cups (500 ml) boiled water, steep for 10 minutes, then drink (you can eat the berries, too).

GROWS/WHERE TO FIND
> can be difficult to get established, then freely sends out suckers to become invasive
> prefers fertile soil
> very salt tolerant
> buy dried berries from natural food stores

Hops
Humulus lupulus

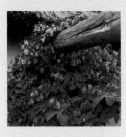

Mild prolonged insomnia can cause real distress, but doctors are sometimes reluctant to prescribe sleeping pills because of their addictive properties. Using hops is a good alternative: It's a gentle sedative with none of the addictive or narcotic side effects of commercial sleeping tablets. You can drink it as tea (but add honey; it's bitter), take it as a tincture (see Using Plants, page 34) or use the dried flowers in a sleep-inducing pillow (see recipe on page 121). (Hops are also used in beer, but the sedative effect doesn't survive the brewing process well; it's the alcohol, not the hops, that makes you sleepy.) The yellow flowers, or strobiles, of hops contain bitter acids and essential compounds that are calming and generally reduce anxiety and nervous excitement. They also relieve tension in the abdomen, thus soothing nervous indigestion. A cup or two of hops tea every day can also help with menopausal symptoms, because it contains estrogen-boosting compounds.

GROWS/WHERE TO FIND
> prefers sunny location
> rampant climber, so provide sturdy supports
> can overwhelm nearby plants
> dry flowers

Kiwifruit
Actinidia deliciosa

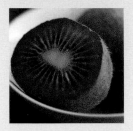

The brown-skinned, green-fleshed, black-seeded kiwifruit used to be called the Chinese gooseberry and is native to China, where it grows wild. The roots, fruits, and leaves of the plant are used in traditional Chinese medicine, but in the West only the fruits are consumed. High in vitamins C and E, potassium, magnesium, and copper, the fruit is eaten or processed for use in beauty products to improve skin and hair.

Kiwifruit have several health benefits: They're thought to have a beneficial effect on heart function and to decrease the amount of fats in the blood. They also contain lutein, which can improve eye health. They're worth eating regularly for their all-around health benefits and can also be mashed and made into a variety of homemade facial-care products (see Kiwi and Papaya Face Mask, page 136).

CAUTION: Kiwifruit can cause allergies, including skin irritation: If this occurs, discontinue use.

GROWS/WHERE TO FIND
> vigorous climber
> likes sun and shelter; for example along a south-facing wall
> needs rich, free-draining soil
> water and feed in summer
> male and female plants needed for fruit
> train as espaliers for best fruit
> prune 3-year-old stems in winter

Lemon
Citrus limon

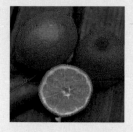

Lemon is one of the most versatile and widely used fruits in the world, primarily as a zesty flavor in cooking. It's high in vitamin C and is often added to cough medicines and lozenges. Applied to the skin, it has antibacterial and astringent effects, which helps to clear up blemishes and brighten dull or oily skin and hair (see Lemon Jelly Peeling Face Mask, page 136). It's also used in many beauty treatments to help with cellulite, though more research is needed in this area. The essential oil, made from lemon zest, has been used to calm and soothe mental fatigue and insomnia, and lift spirits.

As a hair lightener, add the juice of a lemon to ⅔ cup (150 ml) water, mix, then apply as a final rinse to hair. Leave on for 5 minutes, then rinse with water.

GROWS/WHERE TO FIND
> grow in a pot
> likes sun
> prefers a sheltered site with free-draining soil
> water in summer
> fertilize during growing season
> place in frost-free situation over winter
> will fruit all year-round

Milk Thistle
Silybum marianum

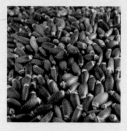

Milk thistle is widely known as a hangover cure, helping the liver when under acute stress and diminishing headaches, skin outbreaks, and digestive problems. Milk thistle is powerfully effective at protecting the liver and helping the body rid itself of poisons. For example, taken before eating the death-cap mushroom, which contains fatal toxins, it's been shown to give complete protection. It is also effective taken within 48 hours of ingesting the mushroom. In Germany and elsewhere, milk thistle is used to treat chronic hepatitis and cirrhosis of the liver but seems to be most effective when used as a preventative rather than a long-term solution to liver problems.

To use, grind the seed very finely, take as a tincture or tea (see Using Plants, page 34), or sprinkle 1 tsp on cereal or in a smoothie.

GROWS/WHERE TO FIND
> biennial
> prefers an open sunny site
> self-sows freely—bit of a garden bully
> need to grow many plants for useful amount of seed
> buy capsules from natural food stores

Papaya/Paw Paw Tree
Carica papaya

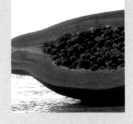

The papaya tree grows mostly in tropical countries, but the fruit is popular worldwide. It's delicious eaten on its own but is also useful to aid in the digestion of protein-rich meals—it contains a mixture of enzymes known as papain, which are used commercially as a meat tenderizer. You can buy papaya enzyme tablets for indigestion or eat fresh papaya with or after meals.

Medicinally, papaya is best known for its use in healing wounds and repairing skin. The green, unripe fruit contains a milky fluid with a high concentration of papain. Applied to skin, it's been shown to help heal burns, slough off dead tissue, improve scar formation, and reduce inflammation and pain. It's used on chronic ulcers and carbuncles, and also for psoriasis, ringworm, and other skin infections. Used in facial masks and cosmetic skin preparations, it has a gentle exfoliating effect (see Kiwifruit and Papaya Mask, page 136). CAUTION: Do not take tablets during pregnancy.

GROWS/WHERE TO FIND
> buy papaya enzyme tablets from natural food stores

Psyllium
Plantago psyllium

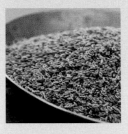

We're used to taking bran as a source of soluble fiber to encourage the digestive process, but psyllium seeds are a better bet, causing less bloating and gas. These tiny, glossy, dark brown seed husks swell up to many times their size to create a gelatinous mass that slowly works through the intestines. On the way, it triggers contractions, scrapes the intestinal walls, and slows digestion, regulating disorders such as diarrhea, constipation, and diverticulitis.

Even more significantly, psyllium seeds have been found to lower the levels of low-density lipoprotein, or "bad" cholesterol, in the blood, thus helping combat heart disease. They also help lower blood sugar levels by delaying the absorption of sugar, and are thus useful for diabetics or people at risk of developing diabetes. They also may help reduce the risk of colon cancer. Adults can take 20 to 35 g a day but should drink lots of water, too.

GROWS/WHERE TO FIND
> annual
> needs sun
> grow outdoors from seed sown in late spring
> buy ready-to-consume seeds from natural food stores

Red Raspberry
Rubus idaeus

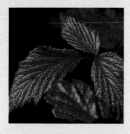

It's the toothed leaves of raspberries, not the delicious summer berries, that are most beneficial in plant remedies. Raspberry leaves were traditionally used during the later stages of pregnancy to ease the birth process (of both humans and animals), make the delivery less painful, and help the uterus get back into shape, but their effectiveness has never been clinically proved. Nowadays we do not recommend that pregnant women take any remedy that has not been conclusively shown to be safe. However, raspberry leaf tea can be used to lighten heavy periods and help combat menopausal symptoms (see also Sage and Raspberry Leaf Tea on page 94).

For Raspberry Leaf Tea, infuse a handful of fresh raspberry leaves in a mug of boiled water. Leave for 10 minutes, then strain and drink.

GROWS/WHERE TO FIND
> prefers sun but tolerates partial shade
> needs moisture-retentive soil
> apply net to protect fruit from birds
> pick leaves throughout growing season
> can grow in most areas

Rosehips
Rosa **spp.**

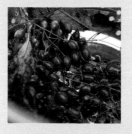

Bright scarlet rosehips are the fruit of the wild (or dog) rose. Although blackberries are quickly stripped from their stems, few people pick rosehips anymore. It's a shame, not least because these tough, hard fruits can be made into a vitamin-rich syrup to keep winter coughs and colds at bay: They contain vitamins A, C and K, plus the B vitamins thiamin, riboflavin, and niacin. During World War II, rosehips were collected by British children and sold to pharmacists to be made into syrup. It's easy to make at home; just follow the recipe on page 76. Strain the syrup well; the tiny hairs (traditionally used as itching powder) are irritating.

GROWS/WHERE TO FIND
> wild roses prefer damp, heavy soil
> fruit found September–October
> take a stepladder when harvesting; they often grow high

VEGETABLES

Artichoke
Cynara scolymus

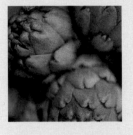

The heart of the artichoke is a culinary delicacy, but the leaves are most beneficial in plant-based medicine, containing a wide range of essential compounds with health-giving benefits for the liver, cardiovascular system, and digestive tract. Leaf extract stimulates bile production in the liver, helping with the digestion of fats, and studies have shown it to be effective for treating indigestion and soothing irritable bowel syndrome.

Artichoke has a double effect on cholesterol: It stops it from being produced in the body and contains antioxidants that prevent the oxidation of low-density lipoproteins ("bad" cholesterol). (See Hawthorn and Artichoke Fruit Leather, page 104.)

NOTE: Consult a physician if you suspect you have abnormally high cholesterol levels. Artichoke should be used in addition to, not as a substitute for, conventional medical treatment.

To make a tincture, fill a glass jar with fresh sliced artichoke leaves and cover with vodka, then seal and leave in a dark place for 3 weeks, shaking occasionally. Strain and bottle. Take 30 drops twice a day.

GROWS/WHERE TO FIND
> prefers fertile, free-draining soil
> needs a sunny spot
> grows very tall, so it might need supporting
> watch out for slugs and snails
> dig manure into surrounding soil in winter
> protect during cold weather
> cut young leaves during the growing period

Celery
Apium graveolens

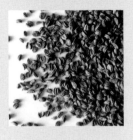

Celery seed was once reputed to be a potent aphrodisiac but nowadays is primarily taken to help with conditions such as gout, anxiety, and arthritis. It's an anti-inflammatory, so it decreases swelling in the joints and is a good diuretic, diluting and flushing gout-causing uric acid more quickly through the system. It also protects against gastric damage caused by painkillers and has gentle sedative properties, relaxing muscles, calming anxiety and aiding sleep. It's probably not worth growing celery just for the seeds (they are tiny, and you'd need to devote a large amount of planting space to harvest enough), but they're easily available in natural food stores.

Celery Seed Tea: Crush 1 tsp seeds and pour over 1 cup boiled water. Infuse for 15 minutes, then strain and drink, up to 3 times a day.

GROWS/WHERE TO FIND
> prefers sun
> seeds ripen August–October
> buy as fresh or dried seed, or extract, from natural food stores and supermarkets
> regional

Chili/Cayenne Pepper
Capsicum **spp.**

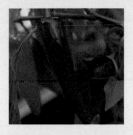

Familiar the world over, chili comes from the U.S., its strongly pungent flavor adding spice to countless dishes. The constituents responsible for the hot, sometimes fiercely hot, impact of chili are also those most involved in its many medicinal applications. It can act as an antiseptic, local analgesic, stimulant, and tonic.

When applied to the skin as a soothant, chili causes a sense of warmth and burning, increasing circulation to the area while desensitizing pain. For this reason, chili is added to lotions, liniments, and salves for muscular aches and pains, resulting in better nutrition to—and clearance of waste products from—the tissues involved.

Chili has antiseptic properties and helps to protect against gastrointestinal infection. It is often added to food in tropical countries to reduce the risk of food poisoning. Used in small quantities, chili helps strengthen a weak digestive system and stimulates appetite.

To make a peppery oil, stir 1 part powdered cayenne pepper into 30 parts olive oil and rub into affected area 3 times a day. Do not use on broken skin. (See also Hot Chili and Mustard Foot Oil, page 70, and Chili Plasters, page 91.)

GROWS/WHERE TO FIND
> tender plant
> grows best in dry soil and full sun
> easily grown in pots

Cucumber
Cucumis sativus

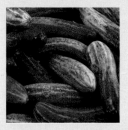

Cucumbers consist mostly of water (with a few vitamins and minerals), so are gentle diuretics and good for intestinal health. They also help to lower blood sugar. But they are included here for their excellent use in topical beauty products for the face and skin. As an anti-inflammatory, cucumbers are often the base ingredient in facial masks, gels, moisturizers, and toners. They have soothing and cooling properties and their high water content means they rehydrate skin, leaving it softer and fuller. (See Lemon Jelly Peeling Face Mask, page 136.)

GROWS/WHERE TO FIND
> hardy
> prefers humid atmosphere
> needs large amount of space for huge root run and sprawling habit
> water and feed regularly
> support stems

Garlic
Allium sativum

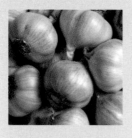

Garlic is a very potent plant: You can smell a large patch of wild garlic, or ramsons (*Allium ursinum*), from many feet away. Extracts from the bulbs are natural antiseptics and are often used in remedies to prevent or combat colds, flu, and bronchitis, and to reduce nasal congestion. Garlic is also known for its beneficial effects on heart health. Studies show it works by lowering cholesterol levels in the blood, especially of low-density lipoproteins, or "bad" cholesterol; by slightly lowering blood pressure; and by slowing arterial plaque formation and clots—an effect that seems to be especially marked in women. Overall, garlic may be helpful in the prevention of thrombosis and atherosclerosis (though with any heart condition, herbal remedies should never be taken as a substitute for medical treatment).

Garlic is also coming under the spotlight for its anticancer properties. A diet rich in garlic appears to lower the incidence of stomach, colorectal, breast, and prostate cancers. Finally, this all-around beneficial plant has significant antifungal properties, which make it an excellent external treatment for athlete's foot (see Garlic Talcum Powder and Garlic Foot Bath, pages 52 and 55), ringworm, and other fungal skin diseases.

For a garlic gargle to combat throat infections, pour 1 cup (200 ml) boiled water over 2 peeled and chopped garlic bulbs. Let steep for 3 hours, then strain and gargle.

Garlic Honey for Coughs: Peel and loosely crush 2 heads of garlic, leave exposed to the air for 15 minutes to allow the active ingredient, allicin, to be formed, then crush finely in a mortar and pestle. Mix into a small pot of honey and leave overnight. There may be a little "juice" on the top; stir in before using. Take 1 tsp for colds, coughs, and sore throats as needed.

GROWS/WHERE TO FIND
- damp woods
- can be grown in pots
- prefers sun
- pick bulbs in autumn
- regional

Purslane
Portulaca oleracea

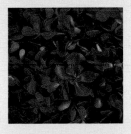

Purslane, an extremely common but pretty weed with fleshy, succulent, lemony-tasting leaves, is well worth cultivating for its unusual health benefits. It is one of the best vegetable sources of vitamin E; glutathione, an antioxidant and detoxifier; and alpha-linolenic acid (ALA), an omega-3 fatty acid obtained only through diet. It's used widely to treat gastric and liver ailments, as well as coughs and arthritis. Although few scientific studies have been performed on it, purslane is used in herbal remedies and eaten as a salad vegetable across the globe—it was reputedly Gandhi's favorite food. Make it into a tonic as a health booster (see below), juice it with carrots, or add a handful of steamed purslane into mashed potatoes.

For a post-viral tonic, gently heat 2 large handfuls purslane leaves and 2 cloves chopped garlic in 2 cups (500 ml) of cider vinegar for 20 minutes. Strain and pour into a sterilized bottle. Take 1 tsp twice a day.

GROWS/WHERE TO FIND
> prefers full sun and dry soil
> not frost hardy
> 2-month growing season
> cut-and-come-again
> can be invasive in warm areas

Watercress
Nasturtium officinale

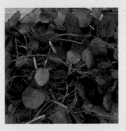

Watercress is one of the most vitamin- and mineral-rich vegetables. It is traditionally offered as a remedy for arthritis and upper respiratory tract infections, and as a general spring "cure," and can also be made into a tonic for the skin and eyes. However, in recent years it's been investigated for its possible preventative effects against some degenerative diseases, including some cancers. It contains compounds called PEITCs (phenylethyl isothiocyanates) and sulphurophanes (also found in broccoli), which encourage cancer cells to self-destruct and builds cell defenses against carcinogens. Research is still underway, but in the meantime, watercress remains a good bet for promoting general all-around health.

As a tea for healthy skin, infuse 1 large handful watercress leaves in 2 cups (500 ml) boiled water and leave for 10 minutes. Strain and drink twice a day.

GROWS/WHERE TO FIND
> plant seeds in a pot with about 3 inches (6 cm) water, and half immerse that pot in a second pot
> or grow in shallow trenches in running water or in boggy soil with light shade
> can cut 10 times a year

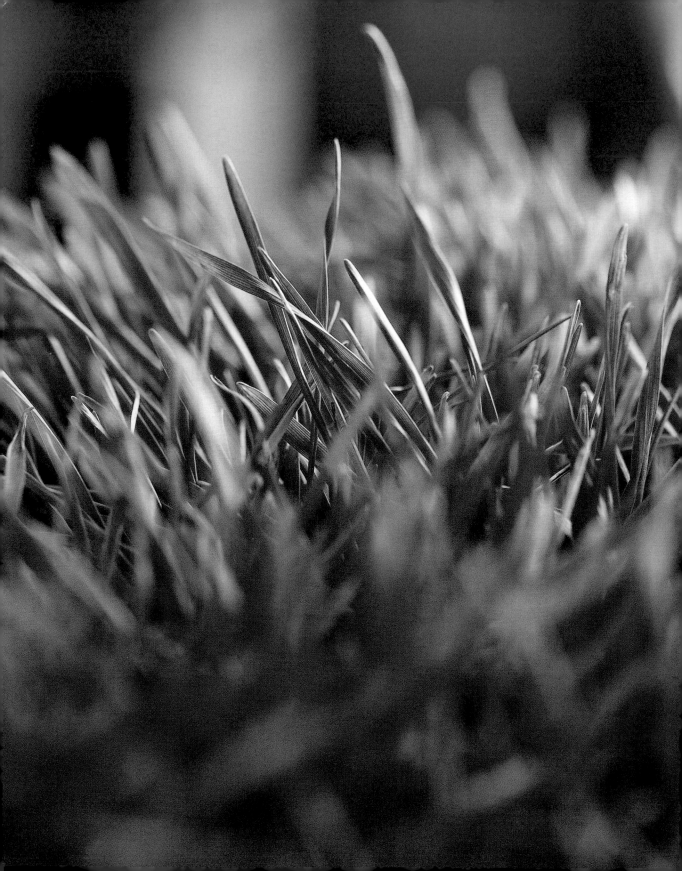

Wheatgrass
Triticum aestivum

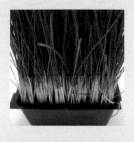

The young, vitamin-rich grass of wheat can easily be grown from seed at home. It improves digestion and has been proved to help treat some diseases of the colon, including ulcerative colitis. It's hard to digest, so juice before using. Some people enjoy the slightly bitter taste, but if you don't, juice with other fruit and vegetables.

GROWS/WHERE TO FIND
> annual, easily grown from seed
> sow in rich free-draining soil in a sunny spot
> can be grown in trays—soak wheat seeds for 8 hours, sow in small tray with compost/vermiculite mix, water daily
> harvest when 5 inches (10 cm) high
> buy at natural food stores

TREES/SHRUBS

Alder Buckthorn
Rhamnus frangula

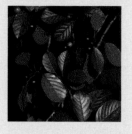

The bark of the alder buckthorn, a small bushy tree, native to northern Europe, gives gentle relief from chronic constipation by increasing fluid accumulation in the gut and stimulating the muscular walls of the colon. Cut a young branch (1 to 2 years old) and strip the outer bark to reveal the papery inner layer beneath. Always dry the inner bark for a few weeks in a cool, dark place before boiling to make decoctions—if used fresh, the active ingredients known as anthraquinones, can make you sick.

For a laxative, simmer 30 g dried bark in 1 qt (1 L) of water for 30 minutes or until halved in volume. Strain, then take 1 tbsp 3 times a day until problem is relieved.

GROWS/WHERE TO FIND
> found in damp woodland and around fields
> a good small garden tree, reaching 16½ feet (5 m)
> protect from strong winds

Eucalyptus
Eucalyptus **spp.**

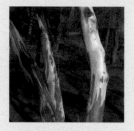

A native of Australia, eucalyptus has long been used by Aborigines as a remedy for colds, sore throats, coughs, and bronchitis. The oil from the leaves works as a decongestant and expectorant and is used widely in over-the-counter cough syrups and sweets. You can make it into a balm (see Pine and Eucalyptus Oil, page 132) for use as a chest rub.

Eucalyptus is an antiseptic used as a topical treatment for wounds and skin infections: Apply crushed leaves as a poultice or soak them in oil and rub in as a liniment. It's also been shown to have a lowering effect on blood sugar levels. Insects dislike the pungent aroma, which makes it a good insect repellent, while herbalists use it as a treatment for bad breath (see Thyme Sweet Breath Spray and Mouthwash, page 41).

To use as a decongestant, pour freshly boiled water over a handful of crushed eucalyptus leaves in a large bowl. Cool slightly, then put a towel over your head and the bowl and breathe deeply.

GROWS/WHERE TO FIND
> found in gardens and wooded areas
> prefers fertile, free-draining soil
> needs full sun
> *Eucalyptus gunnii* is a hardy species (able to tolerate -59°F [15°C])
> cut back to manageable size each year (otherwise grows very tall and branches get out of reach)
> buy oil from pharmacies and natural food stores

Ginkgo
Ginkgo biloba

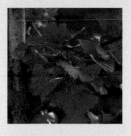

The *ginkgo biloba,* or maidenhair tree, is thought to have been around for over 225 million years, since the age of the dinosaurs, so it's perhaps fitting that its best-documented benefits are for memory enhancement and the mild-to-moderate dementia that can come with age. The dried leaves contain unique substances that are thought to work by improving circulation to the brain, altering the availability of neurotransmitters and enzymes that control brain chemistry and increasing oxygen supply.

Ginkgo has been dubbed the "wrinklies' wonder drug" because it improves concentration, short-term memory, and reaction time in the middle-aged to elderly (see Ginkgo Tea, page 118). It also helps with circulatory disorders, including vertigo, leg cramps, and mountain sickness. By opening up the bronchial passages, it helps with asthma and allergic inflammation and can reduce inhaler use.
NOTE: If you are on prescription medication, speak to your doctor about any counterindications with ginkgo.
To improve memory, make an infusion of 30 g dried leaves with 2 cups (500 ml) boiled water. Leave to steep for 10 minutes and strain, then drink about one cup twice a day.

GROWS/WHERE TO FIND
> slow-growing deciduous conifer
> full sun
> pollution-hardy
> free-draining soil
> harvest summer leaves, then dry before use
> capsule form available at natural food stores

Hawthorn
Crataegus laevigata

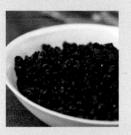

Hawthorn berries are a known tonic for heart health (see Hawthorn and Artichoke Fruit Leather recipe, page 104). They contain compounds that help to regulate blood pressure and heart rate and improve blood flow by dilating the arteries. This helps with circulatory problems such as Raynaud's disease and cold extremities. Hawthorn is also thought to reduce anxiety and mood swings and relieve insomnia.
Hawthorn Syrup: Bring 500 g ripe berries and 2 cups (500 ml) water to a boil, then mash and leave overnight. Next day, bring back to a boil, and simmer gently until the berries lose their color. Strain through cheesecloth, measure the juice into a pan, and add the same amount of sugar. Bring to a boil rapidly, then pour into sterilized bottles. Take 1 tsp daily to help maintain a healthy circulation.
NOTE: If you think you have a heart condition, you must also consult your doctor.

GROWS/WHERE TO FIND
> good as hedging in moderate climates
> white flowers in spring, red berries in autumn
> prune only after fruiting

Horse Chestnut
Aesculus hippocastanum

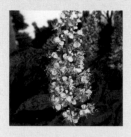

The seeds of the horse chestnut tree are used as a treatment for varicose veins, hemorrhoids and swelling in the lower legs. Varicose veins get twisted and "baggy," damaging the valves that stop from blood running backward, and prohibiting them from working properly. Even more blood then "pools" in the veins, swelling them. Aescin, the essential compound in the extract of horse chestnut, restores the veins' elasticity and improves the flow of blood back to the heart, thus decreasing the risk of clotting and swelling in the lower legs. Horse chesnut can also decrease the likelihood of developing deep-vein thrombosis (DVT) and minimize swelling in the feet and ankles on long flights. (Try the Horse Chestnut Gel, page 88.)

NOTE: Although commercially prepared horse chestnut extracts are taken orally, do not eat chestnuts because they are dangerous when untreated.

GROWS/WHERE TO FIND
> stunning and huge ornamental tree with candelabra flowers
> found in parks and gardens
> collect chestnuts in autumn

Juniper
Juniperus communis

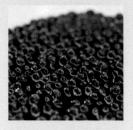

If you suffer from recurrent urinary tract infections, it's a good idea to keep a tincture of juniper berries in your medicine cabinet. The berries take a couple of years to ripen to a dark purplish black, but as soon as they're ready, pick them and soak in oil, or use dried and crushed to make teas and tinctures (see Using Plants, page 34). The volatile oil in the berries—used to give gin its traditional bitter flavor—has diuretic and anti-inflammatory properties, which are helpful with both chronic and acute outbreaks of cystitis. Juniper is also used to treat rheumatism, can gently lower both blood pressure and blood sugar levels, and is often made into an antiseptic balm for irritated skin conditions.

CAUTION: Avoid during pregnancy. Don't use juniper for longer than 1 month, because it can irritate the kidneys.

GROWS/WHERE TO FIND
> aromatic evergreen conifer
> prefers sun
> both female and male plants must be grown for fruits
> collect ripe berries only
> dry on shelves

Lime/Linden
Tilia **spp.**

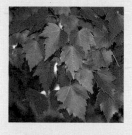

You have to be quick to pick the sweet-smelling blossom of the lime tree: The blooms last for only a couple of weeks in July. They make an excellent dual-purpose tea used primarily to treat feverish colds and flu, but also to calm nervous disorders such as anxiety, irritation, and restlessness. The essential compounds lower blood pressure and have a slightly sedative effect, making this a good drink to have a couple of hours before bed. Children like the sweet taste of linden tea, and it can soothe them when they're overactive or feeling anxious.

To make Lime Blossom Tea, put 3 tsp (15 g) dried flowers in 2 cups (500 ml) freshly boiled water. Steep for 10 minutes, then strain. Drink a little throughout the day.

GROWS/WHERE TO FIND
> easy to grow
> needs moist soil
> short flowering season
> collect buds and flowers, dry in a cool, dark place, then store in tight-lidded jars out of sunlight

Neem/Indian Lilac
Azadirachta indica

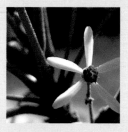

Neem is a large deciduous tree native to India and Southeast Asia. The leaves and seeds are used to treat a variety of ailments, from ulcers and skin diseases to improving digestion and protecting the liver. Like garlic, neem is antifungal, antibacterial, and antiviral, and also brings down temperature in a fever.

However, in the West neem is used mainly as a treatment for head lice and nits—the eggs of the louse, which become "cemented" to the hair shaft. Lice are becoming increasingly resistant to conventional over-the-counter treatments, and neem has powerful insecticide properties, providing a natural treatment that is free of organophosphates. Applied to the hair and scalp (see Neem Nit Treatment, page 79), neem kills live lice. But like all treatments for head lice, it needs several applications to ensure that all the nits have been dealt with.

GROWS/WHERE TO FIND
> can grow in a greenhouse (though it is unlikely to reach a stature where seeds are borne)
> buy from pharmacies and natural food stores

Pine *Pinus* spp.
and Cedar *Cedrus* spp.

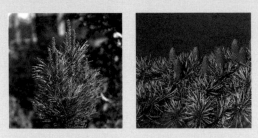

The powerful, "clean" fragrance and decongestant properties of pine and cedar make them popular additions to many over-the-counter cough and cold remedies. The essential oil is distilled from the needles or collected as resin and can be used at home in inhalations, made into a balm to warm stiff or painful muscles, or as an antiseptic deodorant (see Pine Spray, page 135), which kills odor-causing germs and covers unpleasant smells.

As a decongestant, try a pine-needle steam inhalation. Place 1 handful crushed fresh green pine needles in a bowl, and add 1 qt (1 L) boiling water. Then inhale the steam and fragrant pine oil by putting your face over the bowl, taking care not to get scalded. Keep the steam in by putting a towel over your head.

GROWS/WHERE TO FIND
> fast-growing evergreen conifers
> found in wodded areas
> prefers full sun
> needs acidic soil
> inhibit growth of other plants beneath them
> buy resin (see Resources, page 218)

Slippery Elm
Ulmus rubra

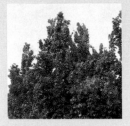

Slippery elm, or red elm, is a U.S. native. It's a fast grower, reaching 197 ft (60 m), and takes its unusual name from the pale orangy yellow inner bark, which is powdered and made into a "slippery" nutrient-rich gelatinous substance by heating with water. (George Washington's army was reputed to have survived on it during the brutal winter of 1777–78). It also has a soothing, demulcent effect on the gastrointestinal tract. For this reason, it is recommended for use with ulcers, colitis, constipation, and other digestive disorders (flavoring it with sugar, honey, or spices improves the blandness).

Slippery elm is added to syrups, lozenges and cough drops to help with sore throats, viral infections, and bronchitis. Coarsely powdered bark can be made into a poultice (see Using Plants page 34) to soothe burns and skin irritations and to draw out infection in wounds, blemishes and boils.

GROWS/WHERE TO FIND
> prefers moist soil
> needs full sun
> suffers frequently from Dutch elm disease, so it is better to buy powdered bark from natural food stores

Spruce
Picea **spp.**

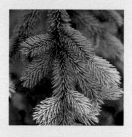

Don't throw away your Christmas tree; it can have healing properties. The traditional Norway spruce, easily grown in pots as well as in the garden, has been found to have antimicrobial properties, limiting the growth of various bacteria. The resin from spruce can be made into a salve (see Using Plants, page 34) and applied to wounds, including blemishes, ulcers, boils, chronic bed sores, and other skin infections. Spruce needles, freshly picked, are also used to make a soothing inhalant for coughs, colds, and flu.

To make an energizing, aromatic bath oil, place a few handfuls of fresh green spruce needles to fill a small sterilized Mason jar. Cover with olive oil and leave for 2 weeks, shaking occasionally. Strain and bottle.

GROWS/WHERE TO FIND
> evergreen conifer
> found widely in wooded areas
> will grow in pots
> prefers damp, acidic soil

Tea Tree Oil
Melaleuca alternifolia

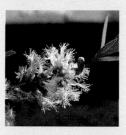

You won't be able to grow a tea tree here very easily outdoors, but the oil is well worth buying and keeping in your medicine cabinet.

It's a natural antiseptic that helps treat bacterial and fungal infections all over the body. The oil, distilled from the leaves and twigs, is marketed as a cure-all and is used in many commercial preparations for acne, skin breakouts, cuts, wounds, dandruff, lice and scabies infestations, bad breath, and thrush. Make it into a balm and use for mild-to-moderate acne. It will help reduce pustules and inflammation without the drying and flaking effect caused by many over-the-counter preparations. It's also effective as an antifungal lotion or cream for topical use for athlete's foot or nail infections if used regularly for several weeks.

As a mouthwash for oral thrush, dilute 3 drops tea tree oil in ½ cup warm water. Swish around mouth for 60 seconds. Spit out. Do not swallow. Repeat 4 times daily.

CAUTION: Do not take tea tree oil internally, and keep away from children. Do not use full strength on skin; it can cause contact dermatitis.

GROWS/WHERE TO FIND
> buy from pharmacies or natural food stores
> can be grown in a cool greenhouse, but more as a curiosity than a plant for oil

Thuja
Thuja occidentalis

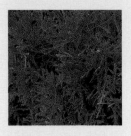

Warts are caused by the human papilloma virus. They generally disappear by themselves, but this can take a long time; two years or more is normal. They're contagious by touch, so it's a good idea to speed up the process if you can. The leaves and branch ends of thuja, an evergreen conifer, have been widely used traditionally to treat warts. It seems to work most successfully on small to medium-sized warts—the large, spreading cauliflower-type warts are harder to treat.

You can also harvest and dry the leaves/branch tips, then make them into a tincture, oil, or balm (see Using Plants, page 34) to use directly on skin to soothe rheumatic pains, neuralgia, and sore muscles.
CAUTION: The essential compound is called thujone, which is toxic when taken internally in large doses. Thuja also stimulates contractions of the womb and encourages menstruation, so it should not be taken internally by pregnant women.

GROWS/WHERE TO FIND
> easy-to-grow evergreen conifer
> prefers moist, deep soil
> grow in a sheltered site
> needs full sun

Uva-ursi
Arctostaphylos uva-ursi

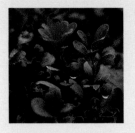

The leaves of uva-ursi, or bearberry, a small evergreen shrub, are used to treat urinary tract infections, including cystitis and inflammation of the urethra. It is often sold in a mixture of herbs as a bladder and kidney tonic tea. Used with dandelion in one trial, uva-ursi was shown to have a signficant effect on recurrent cystitis and has also been used to treat frequent and painful urination.

GROWS/WHERE TO FIND
> small evergreen shrub
> prefers damp, acidic soil
> harvest green leaves in early autumn, then dry

Willow Bark
Salix alba **spp.**

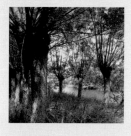

When you take aspirin, you're experiencing the painkilling effect of salicin, the active compound in willow, which is converted in the body to the same compound as aspirin (salicylic acid). In fact, chewing on a piece of willow bark has been a well-known headache remedy for hundreds of years. In trials, the bark has also been shown to have significant success in relieving painful inflammatory conditions such as osteoarthritis, back pain, and rheumatism.

It's best to harvest the bark in the spring. It's worth knowing that the common white willow (*Salix alba*) is less potent than crack willow (*S. fragilis*), purple willow (*S. purpurea*), or violet willow (*S. daphnoides*). With a sharp knife, strip off lengths from young branches, being careful to take only a little bark from each one. You can dry the bark for decoctions or make it into a tincture (see Using Plants, page 34). Use as you would aspirin for pain relief from headaches, menstrual pains, sports injuries, backache, muscle aches, and arthritis. It also brings down fever.

Although willow bark is slower to act than popping an aspirin, the effect is longer lasting. It's also less likely than aspirin to cause gastric problems and internal bleeding, so it makes a good substitute for people with sensitive stomachs.

CAUTION: Be aware that willow bark does not have the same blood-thinning effects as aspirin. Do not take during pregnancy or when breastfeeding.

GROWS/WHERE TO FIND
> deciduous tree, often growing along riversides
> prefers wet/damp soil in sun
> roots are invasive, so don't grow near buildings

Witch Hazel
Hamamelis virginiana

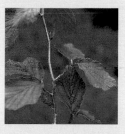

If you want one top performer in your medicine cabinet for everyday family ailments, make it a bottle of witch hazel. The extract of this winter-flowering shrub is the first port of call for bruises, sprains, burns, blemishes, boils, and general skin irritations and can help reduce bleeding when applied topically to wounds. It's highly regarded as an astringent to contract the swelling of varicose veins and hemorrhoids, and is a successful antiviral in the treatment of cold sores (*Herpes simplex*). It can also be used as a soother and anti-inflammatory for sore throats and laryngitis.

You can buy ointments and lotions made from the leaves, and the twigs are steam-distilled to make extract of witch hazel for normal household use. To make a gel to help with the treatment of acne, see page 60.

To make a witch hazel gargle for sore throats, mix ½ tsp leaves and ½ tsp bark with 2 cups (500 ml) boiled water. Leave, covered, for 1 hour. Strain and use to gargle 3 times a day.

GROWS/WHERE TO FIND
> hardy but slow-growing deciduous shrub
> prefers damp soil and sun
> sweet-smelling winter flowers
> use leaves in spring and summer
> buy the extract from pharmacies or natural food stores

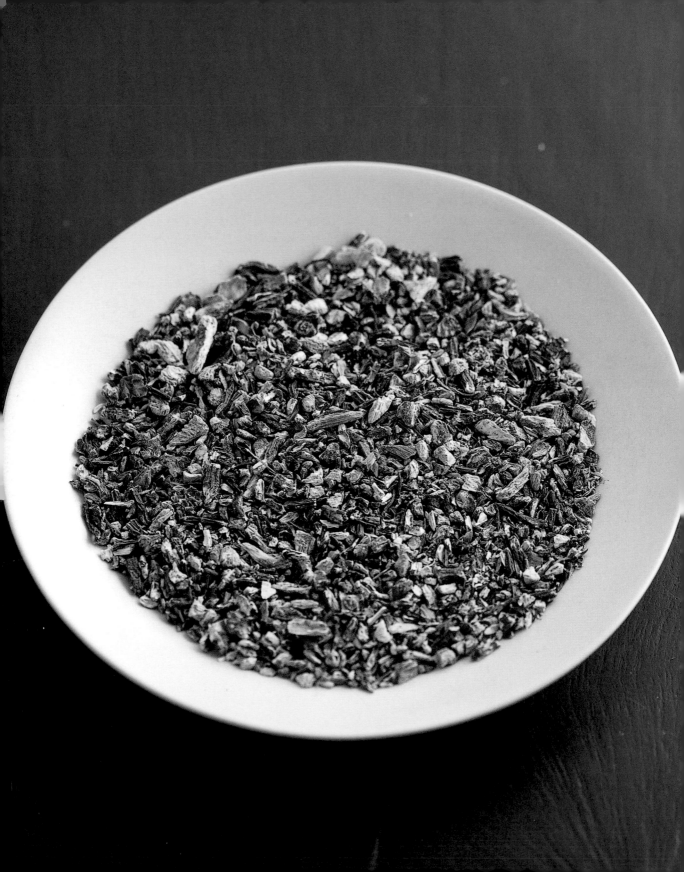

ROOTS

Angelica
Angelica archangelica

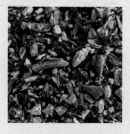

If you know of angelica only as candied green cake decorations or as a flavoring in liqueurs, think again. This common but statuesque plant has many medicinal uses and is especially good in the treatment of indigestion, easing cramps and stopping flatulence. It's also used as an appetite stimulator. It's an anti-inflammatory and expectorant, helpful in loosening up nasal congestion. You can make it into a honey or drink as a decoction (see Using Plants, page 34). It also has a reputation as a "warming" herb, increasing blood flow to the arms and lower legs.

If you are able to pick angelica in the wild, be careful to identify it correctly, because the many members of the parsley family look very similar. The roots are the most powerful part, though flowers, stalks, and seeds can be used, too. Harvest roots in the autumn of their first year of growth, then slice in half and dry before using.

To soothe gurgly tummies, simmer 3 handfuls (30 g) chopped dried angelica root in a pan with 1 qt (1 L) water for 20 minutes (until reduced by half). Strain and drink 3 times a day. (See also Angelica Tummy Soother, page 44.)

GROWS/WHERE TO FIND
> biennial, or to keep as a perennial, remove the flowerheads to stop seed setting
> prefers damp soil
> grows wild
> grows to 6 feet (2 m)
> needs staking
> blooms June–July
> harvest roots in autumn

Black Cohosh
Actaea racemosa

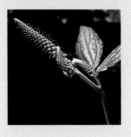

Black cohosh, the bugbane plant, is often taken to relieve the symptoms of menopause, including hot flushes, night sweats, depression, and anxiety. It's supposed to give the benefits of estrogen replacement by balancing the hormones without any of the unwanted side effects of taking estrogens. It's also used to regulate periods and soothe rheumatic and other inflammatory conditions.

Although the menopause-easing effects of black cohosh have had positive reports from Europe over many years, scientific studies have not yet replicated the effects, so more work needs to be done. In the meantime, it may be worth seeing if black cohosh works for you. The plant is easy to grow in gardens, and the root should be dried before making into decoctions or tinctures (see Using Plants, page 34).

CAUTION: Don't use during pregnancy, and don't take for more than 6 months. Blue cohosh is not from the same plant family.

GROWS/WHERE TO FIND
> prefers moist soil in light shade
> nutrient-greedy, so inhibits plants around it
> divide clumps when they get large
> harvest roots in autumn
> rinse roots, then leave for several weeks to dry
> buy extract from natural food stores

Chicory
Cichorium intybus

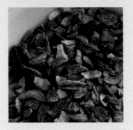

Wild chicory is rather like dandelion: a weed that grows prolifically in many areas with sky-blue, dandelion-like flowers, narrow leaves, and a milky tap root. Both leaves and root are harvested for herbal remedies. Made into a decoction, the roots have traditionally been used for gout and rheumatism, perhaps due to chicory's diuretic properties, and also as a liver protectant.

Chicory seems to provide a broad spectrum of moderate health benefits: Mildly laxative, it's anti-inflammatory and can lower blood sugar and cholesterol. It's a very popular remedy in Turkey and the Near East and is used in Germany as a bitter herb to treat indigestion and increase appetite. You can grow or pick it in the wild and it's definitely worth adding to the pantry. Chicons, the chicory hearts eaten in salads, can be forced from the roots from November onward.

For indigestion, boil 1 large handful chopped chicory root in 2 cups (500 ml) water for 10–15 minutes. Strain and drink to soothe heartburn and acid reflux.

GROWS/WHERE TO FIND
> prefers free-draining alkaline soil
> sow seeds late spring
> needs deep soil for root development
> use leaves before it seeds
> harvest roots in second year; dry for 2 weeks before using

Cleavers/Goosegrass
Galium aparine

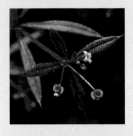

Also known as bedstraw, beggar lice, bur head, catch weed, cling rascal, goose grass, scratch weed, and sticky willy, this is a plant with a history. In medieval times, cleavers was used as a cure-all, but today it is better known as a diuretic, which helps with swollen lymph glands, recurrent cystitis, and other irritations of the urinary tract. The leaves can be infused to drink as a tea (see Using Plants, page 34), but remember to wear gloves when picking—the stems are covered with short, sharp prickles, and the burrs (seeds) stick to everything. Cleavers can also be made into a skin-softening balm.

To soothe scratches, sores, and skin inflammations, pick a handful of leaves (use gloves), crush with a mortar and pestle, and apply directly to the spot, rubbing gently.

For a spring tonic, pick equal amounts of cleavers, dandelion roots and leaves, nettle ends and burdock roots, then wash and place tightly in a Mason jar. Pour over enough vodka to cover. Leave for 4 weeks, shaking occasionally. Squeeze the mixture by hand through cheesecloth, then bottle. Take 1 tsp, 1–2 times a day.

GROWS/WHERE TO FIND
> annual
> grows easily in most situations
> prefers alkaline soil
> pick from the wild rather than introducing to your garden

Dandelion
Taraxacum officinale

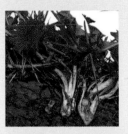

Next time you weed the garden, don't throw out the handfuls of dandelions you may have pulled up. Instead, use them to make plant remedies. Although the root is most often used medicinally, every bit of the dandelion can be used: the flowers in soothing oils; the leaves in infusions (and salads—try them; they're bitter but tasty); the roots as decoctions and tinctures (see Using Plants, page 34). Dandelion is a gentle diuretic and is used traditionally for urinary disorders and poor digestion. Most diuretics leach potassium from the body, but dandelion, apart from being mild, is very high in potassium and other minerals and vitamins, so it also makes a good all-around health tonic. As an oil, dandelion soothes muscles and joints.

To make Dandelion Flower Bath Oil, pick enough fresh flowerheads to fill a small Mason jar. Pour olive oil over to cover, pushing a knife around inside to get rid of any air pockets. Cover and leave on a sunny windowsill for 2 weeks or until the flowers have lost their color. Strain, then pour into a sterilized bottle.

GROWS/WHERE TO FIND
> perennial
> abundant in lawns and fields
> pick flowers throughout growing season
> pick roots in autumn and dry before use

Echinacea
Echinacea **spp.**

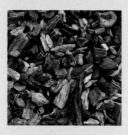

There's not much around that can help treat the common cold, except echinacea. Take it as soon as you feel the signs of infection coming on. Many studies show that it lessens the severity and duration of colds and flu. Try the Popsicle recipe, page 100, and throat spray on page 116.

No one knows for certain how echinacea works, but the theory is that it stimulates the immune system and localizes the infection, slowing its spread through the body. It has best results when used over an 8- to 10-day period after infection, so don't bother taking it as a long-term prophylatic to prevent colds; it won't work. As an antibacterial, echinacea is also used in skin preparations to heal wounds, septicemia, boils, and carbuncles.

NOTE: When growing in a garden, plant *E. angustifolia*: The roots contain more of the known active constituents than the other two main species, *E. purpurea* and *E. pallida*.

GROWS/WHERE TO FIND
> perennial
> prefers sun
> needs rich, sandy soil
> grow in airy, open site (echinacea is prone to mildew)
> harvest roots and rhizomes in autumn
> dry before using in decoctions or tinctures
> buy extract from pharmacies or natural food stores

Ginger
Zingiber officinale

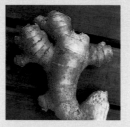

Ginger is one of the most versatile culinary spices used the world over in both sweet and savory foods and drinks. But its primary use in remedies is as an anti-emetic to prevent or control all kinds of nausea, including motion sickness, morning sickness, and vertigo. It's safe enough in moderate doses to be used by both pregnant women and children (see Crystallized Ginger, page 97).

The fresh "roots"—actually, rhizomes, or underground stems—contain essential compounds called gingerols. When dried or extracted, these become much hotter to the taste and also twice as potent. These seem to have a blocking effect on certain types of serotonin receptors involved in sickness, suppressing gastric-acid production and reducing vomiting. This has a soothing effect on the digestive tract and quells stomach disorders like dyspepsia.

Ginger also has a warming effect on the body, and makes a good tea to have on a winter afternoon. It's also thought to be helpful as an anti-inflammatory for arthritic joints and rheumatic pains.

For a warming ginger tea, peel and chop a 2-inch (5-cm) root, then pour a cupful of boiling water over and leave for 8 minutes. Add honey or a squeeze of fresh lemon juice to taste, if desired.

GROWS/WHERE TO FIND
> can be grown at home—choose a budding rhizome (with a little green "horn")
> suspend over water with cocktail sticks until roots form, then plant 4 to 8 inches (10 to 20 cm) deep in potting compost
> keep warm and moist
> likes light shade
> no direct sunlight
> not frost-tolerant; keep indoors in winter
> harvest rhizomes when 1 year old
> not typically grown in North America

Horseradish
Armoracia rusticana

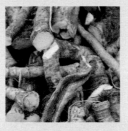

This pungent eye-watering root is traditionally served as a relish with roast beef. Like mustard, it is bitingly hot and has a stimulating effect on the body. It's very easy to grow and has docklike leaves and yellowy-white roots. The edible roots can be made into a balm (see Using Plants, page 34) to rub on to aching muscles or stiff joints, encouraging blood to rush to the area. Horseradish stimulates the digestive system, induces sweating, and clears the nasal passages. It can also be made into a tincture to lessen the severity of colds, flu, and cough.

GROWS/WHERE TO FIND
> perennial
> grow in a large container
> very invasive roots
> harvest roots in autumn
> can grow in most areas

Licorice
Glycyrrhiza glabra

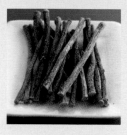

Licorice root is the single most popular ingredient in Chinese medicine, prescribed in many herb mixtures as a harmonizer. In the United Staes, it's a common flavoring in sweets. Licorice is known to loosen congestion in respiratory tract infections and has a long history of use for soothing coughs, colds, bronchitis and sore throats (see Marshmallow and Licorice Cough Syrup, page 103). It's also anti-inflammatory and has slight anti-allergenic properties and is used by some herbalists to help with asthma.

It has anti-ulcer effects, too, so if you suffer from gastric ulcers, try taking a tincture or decoction of licorice or make it into a gargle for mouth ulcers. As a soother or demulcent, it's used for a wide range of stomach disorders, from indigestion to constipation and bowel spasm. In Japan studies have also shown it to protect the liver and have benefits for chronic hepatitis.

NOTE: Take only small amounts of licorice (no more than 20 g a day) for up to 4 weeks.

GROWS/WHERE TO FIND
> perennial
> prefers protected site in sun
> needs deep root run
> grows to 4 feet (1.4 m), so best to stake
> harvest roots from 3- to 4-year-old plants

Marshmallow
Althaea officinale

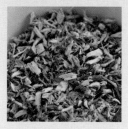

Marshmallow is essentially a gentle soother. The roots and leaves contain a high level of mucilage, a gelatinous substance that can soothe and reduce inflammation in the respiratory, urinary, and digestive tracts. Marshmallow is well known as an expectorant and cough preventer, often found in cough drops and syrups for sore throats and bronchial complaints. The French have used it for centuries in soft cough lozenges, called pâte de guimauve; these bear no relation to the gelatinous marshmallows we eat as sweets today, which contain little if any marshmallow root. As a stomach soother, marshmallow is gentle enough to be used by all ages, especially for peptic ulcers and gastric inflammation. Applied externally as a poultice or balm, it soothes, softens, and heals, reducing inflammation in infected skin complaints such as ulcers, boils, and abscesses.

GROWS/WHERE TO FIND
> perennial
> prefers sun
> prefers moist soil
> needs support at full height
> harvest roots from plants 3 to 5 years old

Turmeric
Curcuma longa

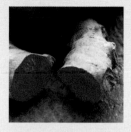

This dark yellow curry plant is widely regarded in India as a tonic for digestive and liver disorders and as a wound healer. It's the active ingredient in "golden milk," an Ayurvedic cure-all.

Turmeric is increasingly being used by herbalists here as an anti-inflammatory for the stiffness and pain of arthritic joints and for skin diseases, either applied externally as a paste or ointment, or taken internally by tincture or decoction. The underground stems, or rhizomes, contain essential compounds that have been shown experimentally to reduce inflammation and also to have a liver-protective effect. However, turmeric is hard to grow in northern regions; it is much easier to use dried powdered root instead.

To make a paste for wounds, put 3 tbsp (30 g) dried turmeric powder in a pan with ⅔ cup (150 ml) water and simmer to a thick paste. Place gauze on affected area and apply the paste for a few minutes, 3 times a day.

To make Golden Milk, put ¾ cup (200 ml) milk, ½ tsp turmeric paste (see above), 1 tsp almond oil and honey (to taste) in a pan. Heat to just below boiling point. Then blend in a blender to froth (adding fruit such as bananas and berries, for taste).

GROWS/WHERE TO FIND
> native to southern India
> tender, tropical plant; grow in pots
> prefers light shade
> keep dry over winter months
> buy as dried powder from supermarkets or in capsules from natural food stores

Valerian
Valeriana officinalis

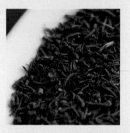

This statuesque plant is well worth planting as a backdrop in gardens for its pink-white flowers and divided leaves. And if you're an insomniac or poor sleeper, there's even more benefit than just its beauty. Valerian is a natural, effective tranquillizer, reducing the time it takes to fall asleep and improving the quality of sleep during the night (see Valerian Hot Chocolate, page 123). It's very safe, with no adverse effects when taken with alcohol and without any next-day problems such as drowsiness and lack of concentration. The sedative effect also calms anxiety, hyperactivity, nervous tension, and irritations arising from stress and can be useful in the treatment of generalized anxiety disorder (GAD).

Make the roots into decoctions and tinctures for daily use (see Using Plants, page 34). Valerian is more effective when taken over a period of 4 weeks and does not have dependency or withdrawal problems. But be warned: It doesn't smell nice.

GROWS/WHERE TO FIND
> easy to grow
> prefers sun or partial shade
> produces more roots if not allowed to flower
> protect from cats, which like to roll in it
> harvest roots in autumn from 2-year-old plants

HERBS

Centaury
Centaurium erythraea

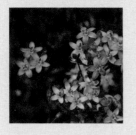

Centaury grows in chalky meadows and grassy banks, but it's an easy plant to overlook: The pink starlike flowers are in evidence from June to September, but they open for only a few hours a day when the weather is sunny. Centaury is from the same family as gentian, and it has many of the same properties as that alpine herb. Once upon a time, it was called "bitterwort" and it is **very** bitter, being used as a flavoring in vermouths and other alcoholic aperitifs. It is traditionally used for disorders of the upper digestive tract, such as heartburn and indigestion, as well as a tonic for liver and gallbladder complaints. Taken before meals, it's believed to stimulate the appetite.

Pick the whole plant during the flowering season and dry before making into tinctures or infusions (see Using Plants, page 34). Sip slowly to allow the bitter compounds to encourage activity in the digestive tract. Freshly crushed leaves can also be used as a poultice for sores and irritations on the skin.

To settle the stomach, take 1½ tbsp (15 g) dried herb and infuse for 10 minutes in 2 cups (500 ml) boiled water. Strain, and add honey to taste (it will be bitter). Sip slowly.

GROWS/WHERE TO FIND
> biennial meadow plant
> difficult to grow in gardens
> plant in wildflower meadow
> prefers full sun
> harvest whole plant and dry for later use

Dill
Anethum graveolens

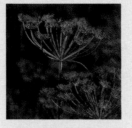

The feathery, flavorful dill leaf is known worldwide as a culinary herb, but the seeds are more commonly harvested for use in herbal remedies. Dill seed has a mild effect and is used to help calm digestive disorders, especially those involving abdominal gas or intestinal spasms. Crushed, then made into a decoction, the seeds can help ease cramping and expel flatulence. Dill seed was traditionally used as a treatment for colic in infants. Chewing dried dill seeds on a regular basis is thought to alleviate bad breath.

To dry dill seeds: When the seeds are ripe and brown on the stem (usually around August), cut the stems off, bunch a few together, and tie inside a paper bag. Hang upside down in a dry, cool, well-ventilated place for a couple of weeks. Shake, and the seeds will drop out into the bag. Store them in an airtight container.

To make a dill seed tea, steep 3 tbsp (30 g) dried seeds in 2 cups (500 ml) boiled water. Leave for 10 minutes and strain, then drink as a stomach soother after meals.

GROWS/WHERE TO FIND
> annual
> easy to grow from seed
> 2 weeks germination (if warm)
> self-sows abundantly
> inhibits the growth of carrots
> seeds ripen July–August

Eyebright
Euphrasia officinalis

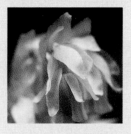

The flowers of eyebright are extremely striking: white with dark purple lines and a central yellow spot. In fact, they look rather like eyes. From the sixteenth century onward, the idea that a plant's appearance offered clues to its medicinal use was very popular—a concept called the Doctrine of Signatures. This is perhaps when eyebright started to be used to treat all kinds of eye problems. There has been little research regarding eyebright's efficacy, but one recent study showed positive results for use in the treatment of conjunctivitis. Certainly, eyebright has astringent properties, contracting and soothing inflamed tissues, which can help with many eye conditions. You can make it into an eye wash (see page 147) or bathe eyes with a soothing eyebright compress. You can even drink it as a tea (see Using Plants, page 34). It's thought to soothe the upper respiratory tract and to be good as a lung tonic, too.

GROWS/WHERE TO FIND
> annual
> found in meadows
> prefers chalk soils
> needs full sun
> grow from seed in moist soil in late spring
> semi-parasitic—its roots feed off neighboring plants' roots
> harvest leaves and flowers while plant is in bloom

Fenugreek
Trigonella foenum-graecum

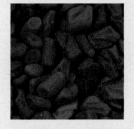

Fenugreek is a native of North Africa and the Mediterranean region and today is widely cultivated in India for use in curry powders, pickles, chutneys, and sauces. The nutritious seeds have a distinctive tang described as somewhere between celery and maple syrup, and are also used in sweet dishes from the Middle East. The seeds contain a high percentage of gelatinous fiber, which accounts for its traditional use as a digestive aid for dyspepsia, diarrhea, and gas. It soothes and relaxes intestinal passageways and is sometimes used to treat gastric ulcers. Fenugreek has also been shown to reduce both "bad" cholesterol and blood sugar levels in people with non-insulin-dependent diabetes.
For glossy hair, crush a small handful of fenugreek seeds in a mortar and pestle, then mix with 3 tbsp natural yogurt. Apply as a conditioner, leaving on the hair for at least 5 minutes. Rinse out.
To make a stomach-soothing tea, boil 3 tbsp (30 g) dried fenugreek seeds in 2 cups (500 ml) water for 10 minutes. Strain and sweeten with honey or sugar.
CAUTION: Don't use during pregnancy, because it can stimulate uterine activity.

GROWS/WHERE TO FIND
> annual
> can only be grown in sheltered sites in full sunshine
> will take 4 to 5 months for seeds to ripen
> buy from natural food stores

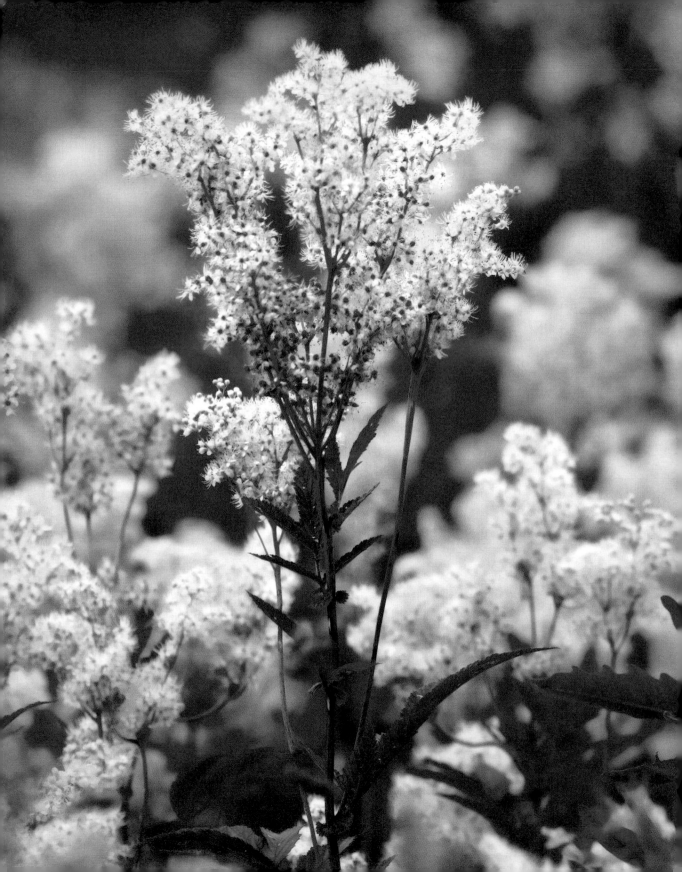

Lemon Balm
Melissa officinalis

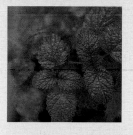

An extremely useful plant to colonize dry, dusty areas of the garden where nothing else will grow. The smell is an added bonus— crush a couple of leaves whenever you walk past to release the tangy lemon aroma. Lemon balm has traditionally been used to soothe nervous tension, relieve anxiety, and promote good sleep. It's also been shown to inhibit the growth of the herpes virus, which causes cold sores (see Lemon Balm Lip Salve, page 108).

To calm anxiety and improve sleep: Make an infusion using 3 tbsp (30 g) fresh leaves, crushed, in 2 cups (500 ml) boiled water. Let steep, covered, for 10 minutes, then strain and pour into a bath before bed.

GROWS/WHERE TO FIND
> grows well in any site or soil
> prolifically self-seeding
> can become a garden nuisance
> cut back aggressively after flowering to produce fresh crop of leaves
> attracts bees

Meadowsweet
Filipendula ulmaria

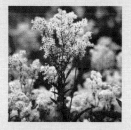

Walking in marshlands or wet woodlands in summer, you'll see the creamy, billowing flowers and tall reddish stalks of meadowsweet everywhere, like plumes of cotton candy on sticks. Harvest the flowering tops on a sunny day, dry them for a couple of weeks, then make into a tea or tincture (see Using Plants, page 34). Meadowsweet is useful in the treatment of acid stomach disorders such as heartburn, indigestion, and gastritis, its antacid and inflammatory properties calming and soothing the stomach.

Meadowsweet, like willow bark, also contains the painkilling substance from which aspirin was developed and has a history of use as an analgesic for headaches. Taken as a tea or applied externally as a compress, it can also help to relieve the inflammation and pain of joint problems such as rheumatism, arthritis, and gout.

For a compress for sore joints, soak a thin cotton cloth in a strong hot infusion of meadowsweet tea. Apply to the joints, leave for a couple of minutes, then refresh.

GROWS/WHERE TO FIND
> perennial
> prefers damp to wet soil
> needs full sun
> found in ditches and marshes
> grow in a marshy patch of meadow or lawn
> dry the flowering tops

Parsley
Petroselinum crispum

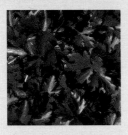

Parsley is one of the most widely grown herbs in western culture, but despite being extremely nutritious—high in protein, iron, potassium, magnesium, and vitamins A, some B's and C—it's more often used as a garnish than an ingredient. It has a strong flavor eaten raw or cooked but is more palatable when made into teas or tinctures (see Using Plants, page 34). Traditionally, all parts of the plant are considered to have medicinal properties, especially the root and seed, which have anti-inflammatory properties. Parsley has been used as a diuretic for water retention and mild kidney and bladder disorders but is not recommended if you have acute or serious kidney problems. It stimulates the kidneys, has an antiseptic effect on the urinary system, and relieves spasms and flatulence in the digestive tract. It's also helpful with anemia, improving iron intake and absorption. Chewing fresh parsley leaves can help sweeten breath by masking other strong odors, especially useful after a garlic-laden meal.

As an insect repellent, the juice from the leaves can be rubbed into exposed areas of skin.

CAUTION: Avoid excessive use of parsley seed and root during pregnancy.

GROWS/WHERE TO FIND
> biennial
> prefers sun
> easy to grow from seed in the sun
> grow in pots
> cut-and-cut-again plant
> harvest leaves before flowering
> use fresh
> buy from greengrocers or supermarkets

Peppermint
Mentha x piperita

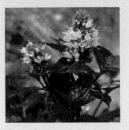

Peppermint has one very unusual effect: At first it's hot to the tongue (the pepper), and then it is refreshingly cool (the mint), hence its name. This hybrid between spearmint and water mint is widely used as a flavoring in food, sweets, cosmetics, toothpastes, and bath products, giving a clean, sharp taste or smell. Peppermint leaves have been used for hundreds of years to soothe digestive problems, including bloating and dyspepsia (see Angelica Tummy Soother, page 44, and "Four Winds" Tea, page 49). Recent studies have shown that it has a very positive effect on the symptoms of irritable bowel syndrome, relieving pain and reducing muscle spasms and flatulence. It also relaxes the esophagus, which helps relieve gas in the upper digestive system through belching.

Peppermint oil is also good for tension headaches. Rubbing a dilute solution of essential oil (not more than 1 part oil to 10 parts water) into the temples and forehead can bring significant relief from headache pain. Peppermint can be found in many over-the-counter cough and cold remedies to relieve nasal congestion.

CAUTION: Don't use the essential oil for infants, either internally or externally.

Relieve nasal congestion with a peppermint inhalation. Put 3 tbsp (30 g) fresh leaves or 3 drops essential oil in a bowl of boiled water. Leave to cool slightly. Place a towel over your head and the bowl and inhale for a few minutes, being careful to avoid scalding.

GROWS/WHERE TO FIND
> hardy perennial
> prefers moist soil
> prefers partial shade
> creeping roots
> spreads rapidly
> grow in pots
> cut-and-cut-again plant
> harvest leaves throughout growing season
> buy essential oil from natural food stores

Plantain
Plantago major

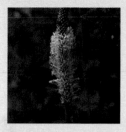

Plantain is one of the best remedies for insect bites and stings. In fact, rubbed onto skin after a sting, plantain—especially ribwort or *Plantago lanceolata*—is thought to be more effective than dock leaves. Plantain decreases swelling and is a natural antihistamine, and a simple poultice of fresh green leaves will help to heal wounds, infections, and other skin conditions. Make a plantain balm to take with you on trips to the countryside (see also Plantain Cream, page 58). Alternatively, use it as a decongestant and expectorant to help loosen coughs and sinuses. You can drink it as a tea (see Using Plants, page 34) to soothe these and other infections of the upper respiratory tract.

GROWS/WHERE TO FIND
> weed
> prefers full sun
> pick leaves at any time and use fresh
> make tinctures from summer-picked leaves
> can be dried for use as tea

Rosemary
Rosmarinus officinalis

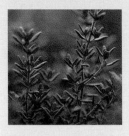

Rosemary is one of the most versatile culinary herbs, an evergreen with a deliciously aromatic flavor often used with fatty meats, like lamb. It's easy to grow in the garden, and you can cut off a sprig whenever it's needed, summer or winter. Rosemary is traditionally known as the "herb of remembrance," and studies show there may be some truth in that claim. It contains compounds that relax the muscles of the digestive tract and can increase the effects of essential enzymes in the brain, thus helping to improve concentration and memory (see Rosemary Wine, page 126).

This stimulating plant can lift spirits and help overcome nervous exhaustion, anxiety, and mild depression. Just smelling it can make you feel better, but to cheer yourself up, drink a cup of rosemary tea or take it as a tincture (see Using Plants, page 34). You'll often see rosemary used in shampoos and conditioners for dandruff and thinning hair, including alopecia, as well as a gargle to sweeten breath.

For a breath freshener, pour 2 cups (500 ml) boiled water over 3 tbsp (30 g) dried rosemary, then cover and steep for 30 minutes. Strain and gargle several times a day. Store, covered, in a sterilized container in the refrigerator.

GROWS/WHERE TO FIND
> evergreen shrub
> needs full sun
> winter-flowering
> easy to grow
> prune in spring after flowering
> in small gardens, try low-growing "Prostratus Group"
> buy fresh herb from supermarkets and essential oil from natural food stores

Sage
Salvia officinalis

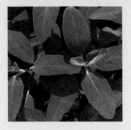

The soft, downy, gray-green leaves of sage don't look as if they pack a big punch. But this aromatic herb has been used in cooking and remedies for over 2,000 years in its native Greece and Italy. It's considered something of a cure-all: Like rosemary, it has a reputation as a memory enhancer, diuretic, and digestive aid and can even help to keep teeth clean (try Sage and Sea-Salt Toothpowder, page 151). But perhaps it's best known for treating colds, coughs, and loosening mucus in the upper respiratory tract. You can use it as a throat-soothing honey (see Sage Honey, page 117) or as a gargle infusion for sore throats, tonsillitis, inflamed gums, and mouth ulcers.

Sage is used to help ease women through hot flashes, night sweats, and other symptoms of menopause (try Sage and Raspberry Leaf Tea, page 94), as well as to reduce lactation. CAUTION: Don't take sage during pregnancy or when breastfeeding.

GROWS/WHERE TO FIND
> evergreen perennial
> can't tolerate wet soil, especially in winter
> prefers sun
> clip back each year to prevent woodiness
> harvest leaves just before plants bloom for drying
> buy fresh herb from supermarkets

Skullcap
Scutellaria lateriflora

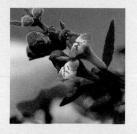

Skullcap is also known as hoodwort, Quaker bonnet, and helmet flower—its hooded violet flowers look like an early military headdress of the same name. It's a U.S. native with a long history of use as a sedative for anxiety, tension, hysteria, neuralgia, insomnia, and other problems of the nervous system. As a natural tranquillizer, it can help reduce muscular tremors and tics, and some herbalists use it to treat drug withdrawal and delirium tremens (the shakes induced by overuse of alcohol). You can make it into an infusion or tincture for soothing nervous agitation (see Using Plants, page 34); take 3 times daily until symptoms pass.

NOTE: If buying seeds or plugs, make sure you get the right species; Chinese skullcap (*S. baicalensis*) is a different plant.

GROWS/WHERE TO FIND
> hardy perennial
> prefers sun
> likes damp site
> moisture-retentive soil
> harvest leaves in early summer and dry for later use

Thyme
Thymus vulgaris

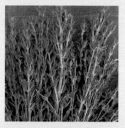

Thyme is a tiny plant, with leaves about 5 mm long and small, dense whorls of white-pink flowering spikes popping up in summer. It's traditionally used in **bouquets garnis** and many meat, fish, and egg dishes. The essential oil contains thymol, which is an antiseptic and expectorant, and is often added to cough syrups and gargles to kill bacteria and loosen phlegm in the throat and chest. Try it as an antiseptic soap (see page 66) for use on sore or infected skin. Made into a salve or lotion, it can be topically applied to help soothe sore muscles and rheumatism. One laboratory study also showed that animals given thyme aged more slowly than others, but this anti-aging effect has not yet been replicated in humans.

CAUTION: Use the oil sparingly in internal treatments because thymol is toxic in large doses.

To soothe aching muscles, fill a sterilized Mason jar with the leaves and flowering tops of thyme, add olive or almond oil, and let steep for 2 weeks. Pour into a bath as needed.

GROWS/WHERE TO FIND
> evergreen perennial
> needs a sunny site—won't tolerate shade
> gritty, free-draining soil
> low-growing
> harvest leaves and flowering tops for drying
> replace after 3 to 4 years if plants become woody
> buy fresh herb from supermarkets and essential oil from natural food stores

Wormwood
Artemisia absinthum

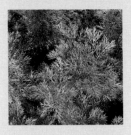

Wormwood is a native British and European plant, which can also grow well in North America. It has deeply cut silvery green leaves, bobbly yellow flowers, and a very bitter flavor. The "bitters" in wormwood increase the production of bile and stomach acids and, taken as an infusion, can aid digestion, ease gas and bloating, and increase appetite. Wormwood is also used as a tincture or tonic to improve the function of the liver and gallbladder.

The leaves and flowering shoots are strong insect repellents (see Pest Potpourri, page 75), which can be dotted around the house, or made into a poultice (see Using Plants, page 34) to reduce swelling from insect stings and other skin inflammations.

CAUTION: Do not use if pregnant or breastfeeding. Do not take internally for longer than 2 weeks because a constituent of the oil, thujone, is toxic in large doses.

GROWS/WHERE TO FIND
> perennial
> prefers poor, dry, free-draining soil
> needs full sun
> prop stems up with canes
> collect leaves and flowerheads in summer for drying

FLOWERS AND LEAVES

Agrimony
Agrimonia eupatoria

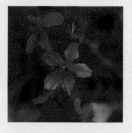

Agrimony has beautiful yellow flower spikes and toothed leaves. It's traditionally been used for liver complaints, including mild jaundice, and its bitter, anti-inflammatory properties can help with digestive problems such as diarrhea and colitis. Nowadays, it's mostly known as a diuretic, which can soothe urinary tract disorders such as cystitis and irritable bladder. Take as a tea or tincture (see Using Plants, page 34) 3 times a day.

For recurrent cystitis, pack agrimony flowers and leaves into a Mason jar and pour vodka over to cover, then seal and leave for 4 to 6 weeks in a dark place, shaking regularly. Strain and bottle. Take 4 drops in water, 3 times a day.

GROWS/WHERE TO FIND
> perennial
> prefers full sun
> easy to grow
> harvest flower spikes and leaves for drying when in bloom

Aloe
Aloe barbadensis

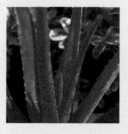

Although aloe is a tender succulent, you can grow it in pots indoors on a warm, sunny windowsill or greenhouse during winter. It's a very handy first-aid remedy for burns, cuts, and skin abrasions—just slice a leaf horizontally and apply the clear gel that oozes out of the center directly onto the wound. Aloe gel has been shown to speed healing time and encourage cellular repair in burns, minor wounds, psoriasis, and the scaly, red, flaking skin of seborrheic dermatitis. It can help skin recover from sunburn and frostbite and is often used in beauty treatments as a skin softener (see Beeswax Lip Balm, page 152). Its astringent properties may also help tighten skin and minimize wrinkles.

CAUTION: The clear gel from the inner leaves is different from the yellowish juice that comes from the tough outer edge of the leaves, which is known as aloes when it has solidified. Aloes can cause intestinal cramping, so don't take orally.

GROWS/WHERE TO FIND
> evergreen succulent
> not hardy
> grow in a pot in a sunny greenhouse or on a windowsill
> feed and put outdoors in summer
> water sparingly in winter
> cut leaves whenever needed and apply gel 2 to 4 times a day

Burdock
Arctium lappa **and** *A. minus*

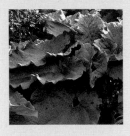

Burdock is sometimes called the "Velcro plant," because the thistlelike burrs stick to anything that touches them. It's a beautiful, tall biennial, and its rosettes of large green leaves are used for infusions and poultices, while its long tap root can be made into decoctions. Burdock has long been used as a treatment for inflamed skin problems such as acne, boils, rashes, psoriasis, eczema, and dermatitis. It's also helpful with the painful joints of gout and rheumatism.

To soothe skin eruptions, steam 2 burdock leaves, drain off excess water, and quickly apply to the skin as hot as you can stand. Cover with a bandage and place a warm (not hot) hot water bottle over the poultice, then leave on for 20 minutes.

GROWS/WHERE TO FIND
> biennial
> flowers June–September
> easy to grow
> use roots in the second spring; they are long and can be hard to dig up

Chamomile
Matricaria recutita

Known more as a pleasant-tasting tea than as a medicine, chamomile can be effective in health problems as diverse as indigestion, colic, inflamed skin, anxiety, and poor sleep. It can be made into a cream for wounds, skin irritations, sore eyes (see Chamomile and Marigold Eye Lotion, page 147), diaper rash and to soothe sore nipples when breastfeeding.

It's also drunk as a tea to help with indigestion, colic, sciatica, and gout. As a mild sedative and relaxant, it can help ease the anxiety and nervous stress that interferes with normal sleep function. Drink a cup 1 hour before bed, or add to a soothing bedtime bath (see Pom-Pom Bath, page 80).

A first-rate remedy for children, chamomile tea can be safely given to infants and children from the age of 6 months upward. For babies suffering from colic and digestive discomfort, breastfeeding mothers can drink the tea. It soothes irritable and overtired infants, gently encouraging relaxation and a good night's sleep. It can also help with the pain of teething.

For a hair rinse, use chamomile tea as a final rinse to lighten blond hair.

NOTE: There are two kinds of chamomile, but the larger flowerheads of German chamomile (*Matricaria recutita*) are more popular in herbal remedies than Roman chamomile (*Chamaemelum nobile*).

GROWS/WHERE TO FIND
> perennial
> poor soil is best
> prefers partial sun
> self-seeds freely
> collect flowerheads and dry

Chickweed
Stellaria media

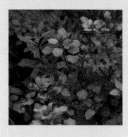

Chickweed proliferates in quiet corners and empty lots, yet its delicate, white, star-shaped flowers are often a welcome sight as the first bloom of the year. It is classified as a weed, but don't be tempted to dig up all your chickweed: This nutrient- and vitamin-rich plant has a wide range of beneficial properties, which are especially welcome during the colder months. Traditionally used in ointments to soothe itching and other inflamed skin conditions, chickweed is also a mild diuretic and, when drunk as a tea, can help with rheumatism. The leaves have a mild, fruity taste and are delicious in salads—treat it as a cut-and-come-again wild green that'll keep your vitamin levels high all winter.

Chickweed Poultice: Mash up leaves or make into an ointment (see Using Plants, page 34) and apply directly to soothe itching, eczema, psoriasis, boils or sunburn.

GROWS/WHERE TO FIND
> winter annual
> weed found in moist soil, beds, and lawns
> blooms late winter to spring
> use young leaves in salads

Cinquefoil
Potentilla reptans

The lobes on the leaves of this common garden weed look like the fingers of an outspread hand— "cinquefoil" is derived from the Latin *quinquefolium*, meaning five leaves. It's an invasive plant with running stems more than 3 ft (1 m) long, and small buttercup-like yellow flowers. Infusions of the leaves and roots have a long history of use in traditional medicine to treat fever, diarrhea, toothache, and mouth ulcers. Cinquefoil has astringent properties; when made into a lotion for the skin, it is often said to help "tighten" tissues for an anti-aging effect. Pick cinquefoil from the wild rather than introducing into your garden—it can spread voraciously.

For toothache and mouth ulcers, infuse 3 tbsp (30 g) fresh leaves in 2 cups (500 ml) boiled water, then cover and leave for 10 minutes. Strain and cool. Use to gargle, swishing around the mouth for 60 seconds, then spit. Use the gargle 3 to 4 times a day.

GROWS/WHERE TO FIND
> perennial
> prefers sun
> invasive, colonizing by runners
> best to pick from the wild
> flowers June–September

Daisy
Bellis perennis

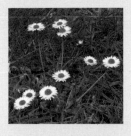

The common daisy is a pervasive lawn invader, so it's satisfying to know that its ever-flowering white-pink blooms can be put to some good use. Daisies have traditionally been thought of as an ideal wound healer and, when made into a salve (see Using Plants, page 34), can soothe cuts, sores, bruises, and stiff joints. Made into an infusion or gargle, the flowers and leaves have long been used to help with all manner of respiratory tract infections, including coughs, congestion, bronchitis, and sinusitis. Daisy tea is also reputed to be a great pick–me-up for listlessness and low energy.

GROWS/WHERE TO FIND
> evergreen perennial
> found in fields and lawns
> prefers sun
> use flowerheads and leaves fresh or dried

Elderflower
Sambucus nigra

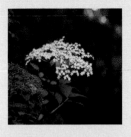

Creamy clusters of elderflowers arrive in June and July and are often used to make cordials and elderflower wine— traditionally drunk hot as a remedy for colds and flu. Elderflowers, like elderberries (see page 161), have antiviral properties that can help combat flu, making symptoms less severe and speeding up the rate of recovery. Take regular infusions as soon as you feel the first signs of infection.

Elderflower is also a good anti-inflammatory and decongestant. Made into a cough remedy, it can soothe sore throats, coughs and bronchial infections and loosen up congestion.

GROWS/WHERE TO FIND
> deciduous shrub or tree, considered a "weed"
> prefers sun but shade-tolerant
> flowers June–July
> use only fresh, cream-colored flowers, before they turn brown

Feverfew
Tanacetum parthenium

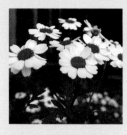

Feverfew has been used to lower fevers and cure headaches since the seventeenth century. But it wasn't until 1974, when a Welsh doctor's wife apparently cured herself of chronic migraines by eating a few feverfew leaves each day that it became known as a treatment for migraine. A flurry of clinical studies followed, and feverfew is now widely used to prevent and lessen the severity of chronic migraines. It can reduce the duration of migraine headaches, decreasing pain, vomiting, and sensitivity to light. Taken regularly, feverfew also seems to make migraine attacks less frequent.

However, the leaves taste very bitter, and some people find them slightly nauseating. You can disguise the taste in sandwiches (see Feverfew Sandwiches, page 122; the butter helps counteract the bitterness) or in a big plate of mixed salad leaves.

For a Feverfew Tea, brew 3 tbsp (30 g) fresh feverfew leaves in ¼ cup (50 ml) boiled water, then cover and leave for 10 minutes. Strain. Drink 1 cup daily, adding honey, sugar, or lemon to taste.

CAUTION: Fresh feverfew leaves can cause swelling and soreness in the mouth. Discontinue if this happens and do not use during pregnancy.

GROWS/WHERE TO FIND
> perennial
> prefers sun
> drought-tolerant
> self-seeds prolifically
> flowers June–August
> use fresh leaves
> for drying, harvest whole plant when flowering

Fleabane
Erigeron karvinskianus

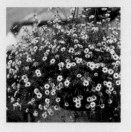

Native Americans burned fleabane to ward off fleas and other pests, which is probably where its common name originated. Today this pretty daisylike flower is a prolific weed, but one with significant herbal uses. It's diuretic and astringent, helping tissues tighten and contract, and has traditionally been used in the treatment of kidney disorders, diarrhea, and menstrual problems. One study showed that fleabane lowered blood pressure temporarily in animals, and it has been used to help stop the flow of blood in minor hemorrhages such as nosebleeds. The leaves and flowers can be infused and drunk as a tea (see Using Plants, page 34).

Fleabane Pet Bedding: Dry leaves and flowers, then crumble and put in a small cheesecloth bag. Place among your pet's bedding. Worth a try!

GROWS/WHERE TO FIND
> annual and perennial weed
> prefers light soils and sunny spots, as well as rock gardens
> bountiful daisylike flowerheads from spring to autumn
> use leaves and flowers

Honeysuckle
Lonicera periclymenum

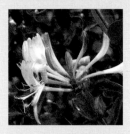

One of the most fragrant garden plants, honeysuckle is also used as a remedy for respiratory illnesses. The flowers are rich in salicylic acid, which has painkilling properties, and can be helpful with sore throats, headaches, bronchial complaints, croup, rheumatism, and arthritis. Drink as a tea or gargle with it for best results. It's also a cooling plant and can calm fever, hot flushes, and sunstroke.

Honeysuckle Honey: Place washed flowers and buds in a jar, leaving a 1-inch (2-cm) gap at the top. Cover completely with honey, then seal and leave to steep for 2 weeks (check that the flowers are always covered to prevent mold). Strain and bottle in a sterilized container. Take 2 tsp a day.

GROWS/WHERE TO FIND
> deciduous shrub
> prefers dappled shade
> prone to mildew (don't allow to dry out, as mildew will set in)
> climber that needs support
> flowers June–August
> use flowers fresh or dried

Lady's Mantle
Alchemilla xanthochlora

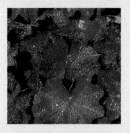

The contrast of the acid-yellow flowers and dark green leaves of lady's mantle make it a stunning groundcover plant in cottage-type gardens. When it blooms from June to September, cut the flowering stems and leaves and dry for use in herbal remedies. Lady's mantle contains essential compounds that, applied externally to wounds, stop bleeding by clotting the blood. You can make it into a salve for use with cuts and wounds, and it's also helpful for stopping general itchiness of the skin.

Made into a tea, lady's mantle is often used to combat excessive menstrual bleeding and diarrhea. Its coagulant properties appear to decrease menstrual blood flow and vaginal discharge after a few weeks' use. The tea can also be used as a mouthwash for bleeding gums, especially after dental procedures.

To alleviate heavy menstrual bleeding, make an infusion with 3 tbsp (30 g) dried leaves and flowering stems in 2 cups (500 ml) boiled water. Cover and leave to steep for 10 minutes. Drink a cup 3 times a day.

GROWS/WHERE TO FIND
> perennial
> slow growing
> good groundcover
> prefers dappled sun
> flowers June–September
> harvest leaves and flowering stems for drying

Lavender
Lavandula angustifolia

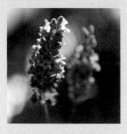

Lavender has been used in bathing since Roman times; in fact, the Latin *lavare,* from which lavender takes its name, means "to wash." With its powerful but calming scent, lavender is now used in a wide range of perfumes, cosmetics, and soaps. The essential oil in the flowers has a soothing, sedative effect, which calms nerves, relaxes muscles, eases anxiety and helps promote sleep. You can use it simply for its scent or in baths (see Lavender Bath Bomb, page 139), or make it into a gently antiseptic salve for cuts and bruises, to help minimize scarring and relieve skin irritations.

Taken as a tea or tincture (see Using Plants, page 34), lavender has soothing effects on the central nervous system generally. It's thought to slow nerve reactions, slightly easing pain and irritability and clearing the mind of nervous tension. It can help with sleeping difficulties; a cup of lavender tea about 1 hour before bed acts as a mild sedative for insomnia. Lavender also aids digestion, relieving intestinal spasms and quelling "nervous" stomach complaints.

GROWS/WHERE TO FIND
> evergreen shrub
> needs full sun
> prefers poor, gritty soil
> good for pots
> for drying, harvest flowers from mid- to late summer, when petals are just opening
> clip back after flowering; don't cut into old wood
> buy lavender essential oil from natural food stores

Marigold
Calendula officinalis

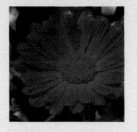

The bright orange marigold may no longer be a very fashionable flower, but it's still extremely useful medicinally, having antiseptic and anti-inflammatory properties and a wealth of potential uses. As a lotion, cream, or ointment, it will speed up healing and counter infection in conditions as diverse as minor burns and sunburn, insect bites and stings, sore and pustular blemishes, acne (see Marigold, Lavender and Rose Geranium Gel, page 64), cuts and abrasions, inflamed rashes such as diaper rash, and hemorrhoids and varicose veins.

Taken as a tea or tincture (see Using Plants, page 34), it helps soothe stomach disorders and ulcers and is also used in the treatment of extremely painful periods, known as dysmenorrhea. Only the flowerheads are used: Harvest them as they bloom.
NOTE: When using marigolds, it is important to choose plants from the genus known as *Calendula*. Trickily in horticulture, most "marigolds" are actually from an entirely different species, known as *Tagetes*. If in doubt check with your supplier, because the medicinal properties of the two species are very different.

GROWS/WHERE TO FIND
> annual
> easy to grow from seed and available as plants early in summer bedding season
> prefers full sun
> good in containers and window boxes
> harvest flowers; deadhead regularly to keep plants flowering

Motherwort
Leonurus cardiaca

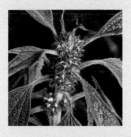

The tall, raggedy, sometimes fluffy flowering stems of motherwort are easy to grow in the garden and, at 5 ft (1.5 m) tall, makes an interesting addition at the back of a herbaceous border. The flowering stems are traditionally used as a heart tonic, the plant's slightly sedative effect soothing palpitations and nervous irritability. It doesn't make you drowsy, just calmer and more relaxed.

Motherwort, as you can guess from the name, has also been used with premenstrual syndrome, to minimize pain, bloating, anxiety, and irritability. It contracts the womb and improves blood flow, so it can be used to hurry along late periods. However, it shouldn't be used by women who already have heavy bleeds or those who may have an underlying undiagnosed disorder. Motherwort can be taken as a tea, but it doesn't taste pleasant. Try it as a tincture or make into a honey instead (see Using Plants, page 34).

CAUTION: Do not use during pregnancy.

GROWS/WHERE TO FIND
> grows easily from seed
> prefers poor soil
> harvest flowering stems in August when in full bloom

Mullein
Verbascum thapsus

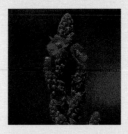

This statuesque plant has long been a staple in herbal medicine, used as an expectorant, decongestant, and mucus reducer for catarrh and to ease chest complaints such as bronchitis. The leaves, made into a lotion or ointment, aid wound healing and soothes inflammation, and the infused oil makes an excellent treatment for earache caused by compacted wax (see Wax-Dissolving Drops, page 82). Mullein's dramatic spiked yellow flowers and felted greenish silver rosettes of foliage look fantastic in any garden. Collect wild seeds or buy and scatter during spring/autumn.

Mullein Tea: Pick 5 to 6 large green leaves during the flowering season (the small hairs on the leaves can irritate the skin, so wear gardening gloves). Wash, then chop and place in a teapot. Add 2 cups (500 ml) hot water and let steep for 10 minutes. Strain. Drink for irritations of throat and chest.

GROWS/WHERE TO FIND
> grows in gardens
> biennial, dying back after 2 years
> best in free-draining soil
> prefers full sun
> self-seeds easily
> flowers early summer
> may need staking

Nasturtium
Tropaeolum majus n

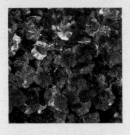

These colorful flowers have a surprisingly zingy flavor and are used to brighten up the look *and* taste of summer salads. Nasturtium has other benefits, too: The flowers and leaves have antimicrobial properties and are used to treat bronchitis, catarrh, and bacterial infections of the upper respiratory tract. The plant's active compounds seem to help loosen and clear phlegm, making breathing easier. Nasturtium can be made into a tincture, honey, or vinegar (see Using Plants, page 34). As a tea, it can be drunk, used as a gargle for infected throats, or as a gentle antiseptic face wash for blemish-prone skin.

To ease congestion, try nasturtium vinegar. Place 1 cup flowers/leaves in a bottle with 1 garlic clove, then pour over 2 cups (500 ml) cider vinegar to cover completely (otherwise the flowers may get moldy). Seal and leave for 4 weeks. Strain, bottle and take 1 tsp twice a day.

GROWS/WHERE TO FIND
> annual
> can be grown in containers
> prefers sun
> self-seeds readily
> harvest leaves and flowers in summer and use fresh

Nettle
Urtica dioica

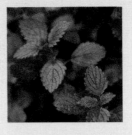

The stinging nettle might not be the most loved plant, but it's certainly one of the most useful. Nettle leaves are very nutritious, high in vitamins, minerals, and chlorophyll. When made into soups or eaten raw (be brave, but roll them up in a tight ball first), they can give the immune system a boost at any time of year (see Nettle Soup and Pesto, page 114). They contain anti-inflammatories and natural painkillers and have a long history of treating rheumatic disorders and arthritis. Recent research illustrates the point: Applied as a lotion to sore joints or drunk as a tea, nettles appear to reduce the pain of arthritis and lessen the need for painkillers, like aspirin and ibuprofen.

The yellow roots provide treatment for an enlarged prostate, a condition that affects many men in midlife. After taking nettle root extract for a few months, both urine flow and frequency were shown to improve.

You can also add a nettle rinse to your hair-care routine to treat dandruff, improve growth, and bring a healthy, glossy shine to hair (see page 128).

To ease the pain of acute arthritis, steep 5 tbsp (50 g) fresh young nettle tops in 2 cups (500 ml) boiled water. Cover and leave for 10 minutes. Strain. Makes 3 cups to be drunk over the day.

GROWS/WHERE TO FIND
> in wasteland, banks, open land, woods
> prefers nitrogen-rich soil
> harvest the top 5 or 6 inches (15 cm) of young tops in spring (wear gloves)
> tops will quickly regrow and can be cut again throughout season
> harvest roots in autumn
> buy root extract from natural food stores

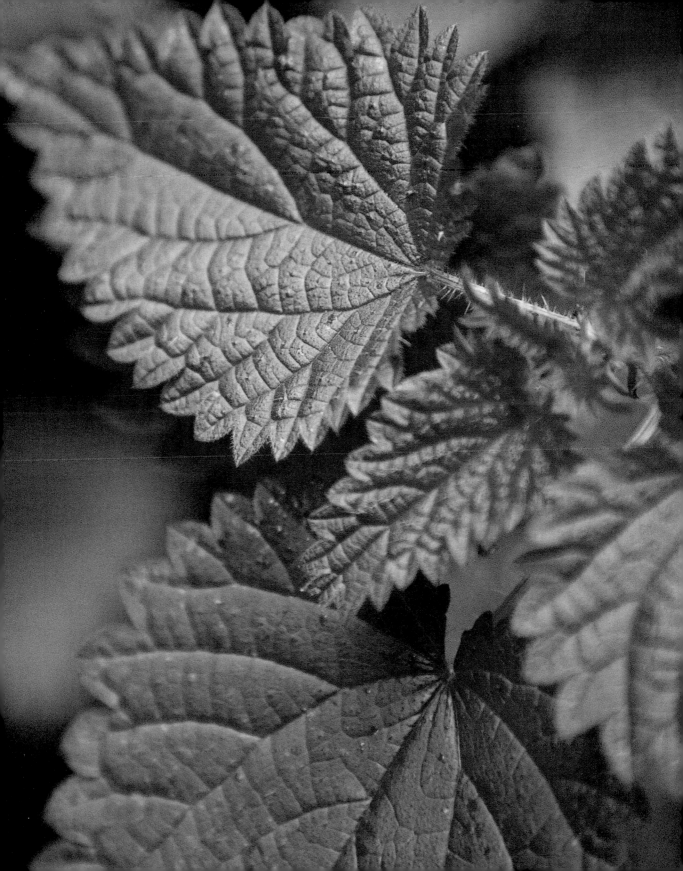

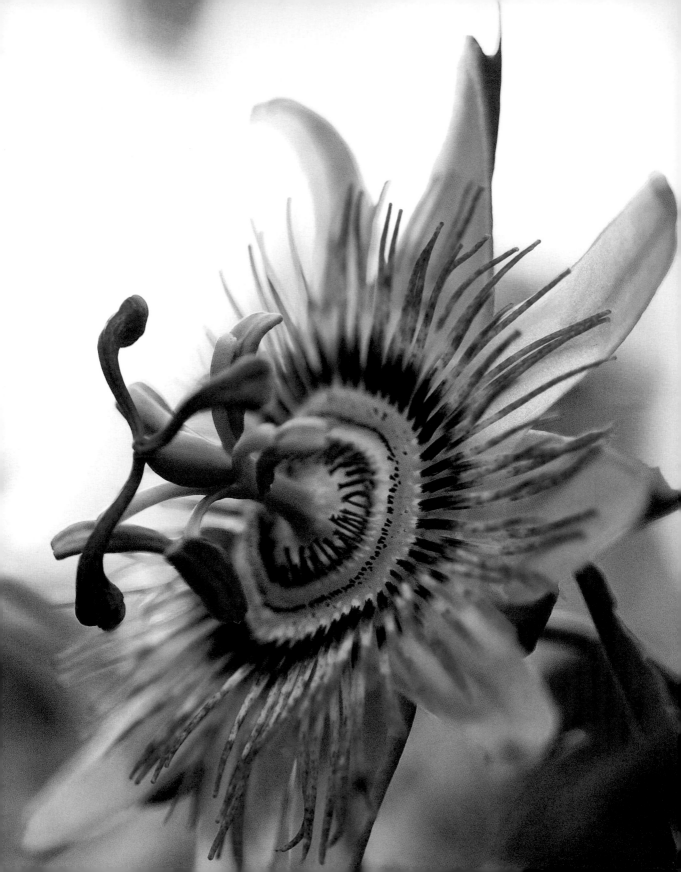

Passionflower
Passiflora **spp.**

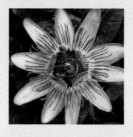

The dramatic showy blooms of passionflower and its leaves have a calming, sedative effect when made into teas and tinctures. Passionflower is often used to treat anxiety, soothe tension and restlessness, lower blood pressure, and help with sleeping problems arising from nervous distress. It can also help settle nervous stomach disorders.

For Passionflower Tea, infuse a few leaves or flower petals in freshly boiled water and drink as a tea 3 times a day.

GROWS/WHERE TO FIND
> climber
> prefers poor, sandy soil
> will grow outdoors in a sunny, protected site
> in colder locations, grow in a greenhouse
> restrict roots to encourage fruiting
> provide support
> use flowers fresh or dried

Red Clover
Trifolium pratense

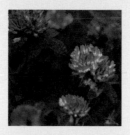

Red clover is found in the wild and used by farmers as a soil enhancer and forage crop. In recent years the flowers have received a lot of attention as a natural form of hormone replacement therapy as a result of menopause. Red clover is high in isoflavones, phytestrogenic compounds that are thought to help reduce hot flushes, night sweats, and other symptoms of menopause, as well as premenstrual syndrome (PMS). But as yet, no major clinical studies have confirmed its usefulness for either menopause or PMS.

Red clover is best taken as a tea made from the dried flowers (see Using Plants, page 34).

GROWS/WHERE TO FIND
> perennial
> found in meadows, paths, woods
> prefers loamy soil
> easy to grow
> harvest open flowerheads for drying

Rose Geranium
Pelargonium graveolens

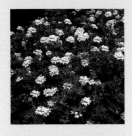

This tender, rose-scented geranium isn't frost-hardy and won't last long outside, but it can be potted and kept indoors in a cool, light room or greenhouse. It's worth it for the wonderful aroma—the essential oil has slightly minty undertones and is very popular in aromatherapy—and both flowers and leaves can be dried and used in potpourri.

In remedies, rose geranium is often used as a balm to soothe acne (see Marigold, Lavender, and Rose Geranium Gel, page 64), eczema, and other skin conditions. It has antiseptic and anti-inflammatory properties and was traditionally used as a tea or tincture to treat nausea, tonsillitis, and poor circulation. Pour the infusion (see Using Plants, page 34) into the bath to soothe skin—you'll definitely come out smelling like roses.

GROWS/WHERE TO FIND
> evergreen shrub
> pot and keep indoors
> water sparingly
> cut back annually to stop plants from becoming leggy
> harvest fresh leaves all year
> buy essential oil from natural food stores

Self-Heal
Prunella vulgaris

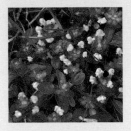

You find this pretty, low-growing plant in meadows and woods, its intensely violet flowers on spikes, with two bracts looking almost like a collar underneath. It's renowned as a wound healer, calming inflammation and helping to stop blood flow, hence its other names: heal-all, woundwort, and hock heal. Make it into a salve for first-aid use on cuts, burns, bruises, ulcers, bites, cold sores (see below) and minor injuries.

Self-heal also has antiviral properties and, taken internally as a tea or tincture (see Using Plants, page 34), can help with throat infections, flu, and fever. It's been shown to hinder the ability of some viruses (including the cold-sore virus) to replicate. The tea can also be used as a gargle for inflamed gums, mouth ulcers, and to soothe sore throats.

For a skin soother, pack a sterilized Mason jar with fresh self-heal flowers and leaves, and pour over enough olive oil to cover. Seal and leave on a sunny window ledge for 3 to 4 weeks or until all color has leached from the plants. Strain, then bottle. Apply to affected area twice daily, or use as a bath oil.

GROWS/WHERE TO FIND
> groundcover perennial
> invasive by creeping underground stems
> grow in wildflower meadow
> cut flowering stems in summer for drying

St.-John's-Wort
Hypericum perforatum

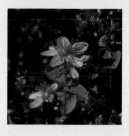

The yellow flowers of St.-John's-wort provide a natural antidepressant. The herb has been used for centuries to treat the age-old disorders of melancholy and hysteria. But in the past thirty years it's been proved as effective in the treatment of mild to moderate depression as prescribed antidepressants—and without many of the side effects. The plant contains hypericin and hyperforin, active compounds that help relieve anxiety, depression, nervous tension, seasonal affective disorder (SAD), and insomnia. Make the flowers into a tea or tincture (see Using Plants, page 34) and take daily.

St.-John's-wort also has a very long history of use as a wound healer. When made into a salve, its anti-inflammatory properties help soothe cuts, bruises, and inflamed skin (see Jelly Balm, page 73). It's also known as an antiviral, which can help with herpes and hepatitis.

CAUTION: Do not take St.-John's-wort without checking with your doctor or pharmacist if you are on any medication, particularly birth-control pills, antidepressants or warfarin.

GROWS/WHERE TO FIND
> perennial
> prefers sun
> good meadow plant
> self-seeds profusely
> summer-flowering
> harvest flowering tops and use fresh or dry
> buy capsules or tincture at natural food stores

Vervain
Verbena officinalis

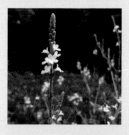

It's unusual to see the delicate, lilac flowering spikes of vervain in the wild nowadays, but it's so pretty and reputed to be such a cure-all that it's definitely worth growing in the garden. Like self-heal, it has an astonishing range of applications and is used for insomnia, depression, headaches, hot flushes, coughs, chronic fatigue, and problems with digestion. It's perhaps most useful as a nerve soother, restoring calm after periods of nervous tension or physical exhaustion, and thus helping to improve sleep and lift mood. It can make you sweat, so it is often used to bring down temperature, and has anti-inflammatory and painkilling properties, so it can help with headaches and premenstrual syndrome. Its bitter and laxative properties make it useful for digestive problems. Take as an infusion made from fresh or dried flowering stems and leaves (see Using Plants, page 34). It can also be applied to the skin to treat burns, inflammation, and wounds.

GROWS/WHERE TO FIND
> perennial
> prefers lime soil
> harvest late in the flowering season for drying

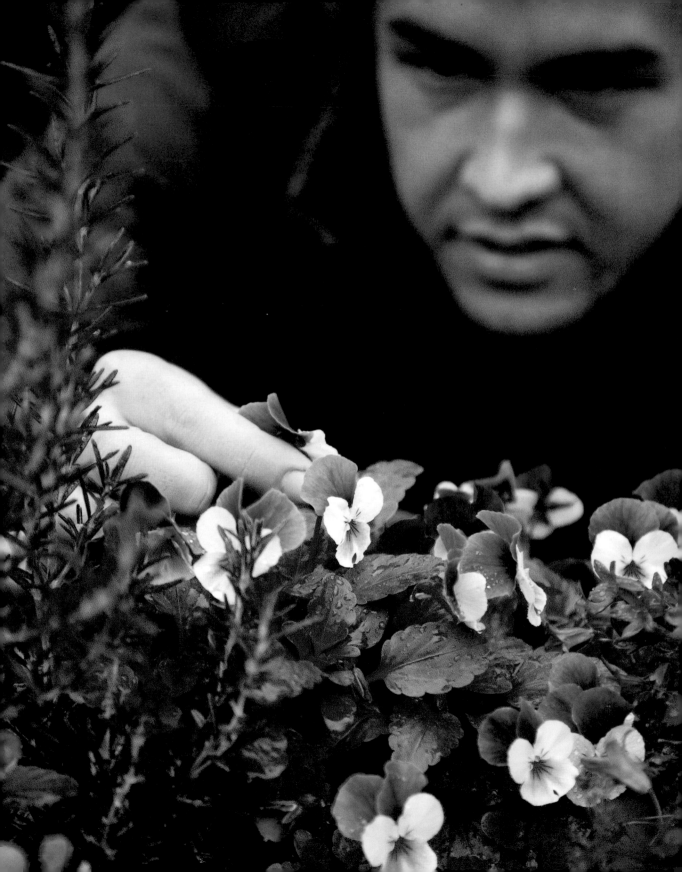

Viola/Johnny-Jump-Ups
Viola tricolor

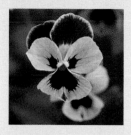

Known as hearts-ease or wild pansy, this tiny plant is cultivated in gardens for its long flowering season. It is an anti-inflammatory and has traditionally been used as a soothing balm for eczema (see Viola and Chamomile Cream, page 56), acne, pustular spots, and other skin outbreaks. Taken as a tea (see Using Plants, page 34), it can loosen congestion in bronchitis and coughs, and its diuretic properties also help with cystitis, rheumatism, and urinary disorders.

GROWS/WHERE TO FIND
> small perennial often treated as an annual
> easy to grow from seed
> prefers partial shade
> flowers April–September
> harvest throughout flowering season and use fresh or dried

Woodruff
Galium odoratum

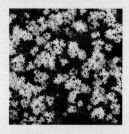

This woodland plant, which can be grown in moist garden patches, smells of freshly mown hay—an aroma that only intensifies when the flowering parts are dried. It makes a delicious tea (see Using Plants, page 34), which is traditionally used as a tonic to boost liver function and help with arthritis. It's a mild sedative and can soothe agitation, restlessness, and anxiety, helping to improve sleep disorders and insomnia.

GROWS/WHERE TO FIND
> perennial
> good groundcover
> prefers moist soil
> tolerates shade
> invasive
> flowers late spring/early summer
> harvest just before flowering and use dried for best flavor

Yarrow
Achillea millefolium

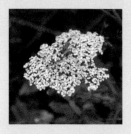

Yarrow is also known as woundwort, nosebleed, staunchweed, and bloodwort; it was traditionally packed into open wounds to staunch bleeding. As a salve or lotion (see Using Plants, page 34), it can be used to stop bleeding cuts and wounds and to improve the healing of bruises, rashes, and hemorrhoids.

Versatile yarrow has many other medicinal properties, too. Drunk as a hot tea, it brings down temperature and encourages sweating, so it is helpful for colds, flu, congestion, rheumatism, and fever. The essential oil can be made into a chest rub for bronchial complaints and coughs. The tea has a bitter astringency (add sugar to taste), which helps soothe digestion and stop diarrhea. Yarrow can also lower blood pressure slightly and, as it contains the painkiller salicylic acid, is useful for headaches, menstrual cramps, and arthritis pain.

CAUTION: Don't use during pregnancy.

To staunch nosebleeds, bruise and roll a few fresh yarrow leaves into a ball and place inside the affected nostril. Gently remove once bleeding has stopped.

GROWS/WHERE TO FIND
> perennial
> grows wild in meadows
> easy to grow
> prefers sun
> flowers June–September
> harvest flowers and leaves while in bloom for drying
> buy essential oil or capsules from natural food stores

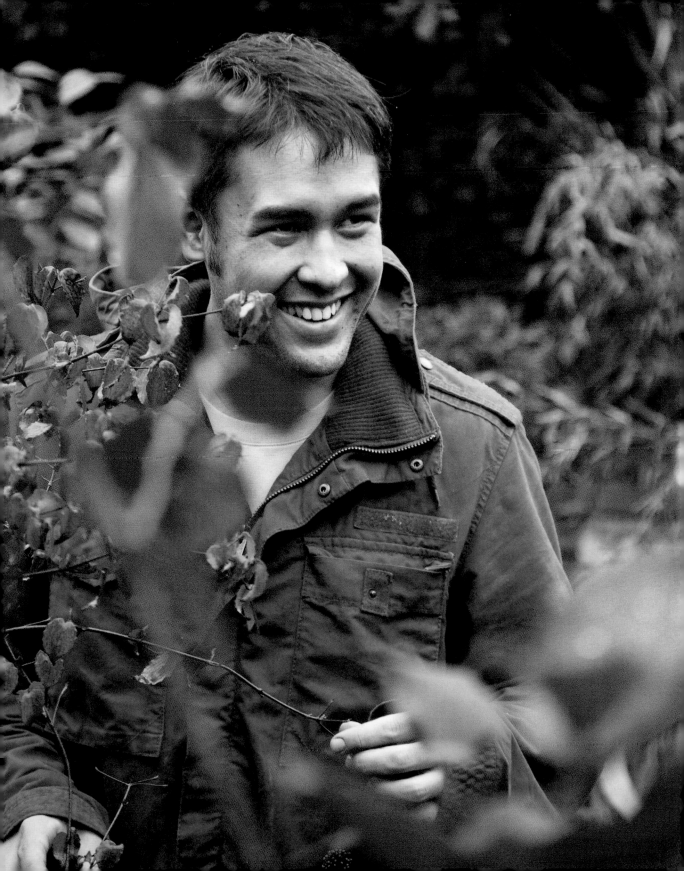

RESOURCES

SUPPLIERS

The equipment and materials you will need to make the recipes are available in kitchen, health-food, and garden-supply stores. Here are a few suppliers that stock more specialized items. These are listed by country but many will ship internationally.

In the United States

CAPRILANDS
Coventry, Connecticut
(860) 742-7244
www.caprilands.com
Nursery and online store

HERBAL REMEDIES
322 7th Avenue, 3-F
New York, New York
www.herbalremedies.com
Online store

MORNING SUN HERB FARM
Vacaville, California
(707) 451-9406
www.morningsunherbfarm.com
Nursery and online store

MOUNTAIN ROSE HERBS
(800) 879-3337
www.mountainroseherbs.com
Online store; essential oils, beeswax and emulsifying wax

MRS. MANGO & COMPANY
3500 South U.S. Hwy. 1
Rockledge, Florida
www.mamaherb.com
Online store

NATURE HILLS NURSERY
Omaha, Nebraska
(402) 934-8116
www.naturehills.com
Nursery and online store

OREGON'S WILD HARVEST
(503) 668-7713
www.oregonswildharvest.com
Stores and online; bulk organic herbs

PACIFIC BOTANICALS
4840 Fish Hatchery Road
Grants Pass, Oregon
www.pacificbotanicals.com

SPECIALTY BOTTLE
(206) 382-1100
www.specialtybottle.com
Online store; bottles and jars

STOKES SEEDS
(800) 396-9238
www.stokesseeds.com
Online store; United States branch based in Morristown, New Jersey

WELL-SWEEP HERB FARM
Port Murray, New Jersey
(908) 852-5390
www.wellsweep.com
Nursery and online store; herbs are available each year after about May 15; website also offers some gardening advice

WILD WEEDS
(707) 840-0776
www.wildweeds.com
Online store; bulk herbs, essential oils, drop/spray bottles, jars, funnels

In Canada

THE CONTAINER STORE
(888) CONTAIN
www.containerstore.com
Online store; bottles and jars,
specialized dispensers

GREEN SPACE DESIGN ORGANIC SEEDS
Cortes Island, British Columbia
(250) 935-0135
www.organic-seeds.ca
Online store; comprehensive selection of
organic flower, herb and vegetable seeds

HORTICO NURSERIES
Waterdown, Ontario
(905) 689-6984
www.hortico.com
Nursery and online store

RICHTERS HERBS
(905) 640-6677
www.richters.com
Online store; medicinal, culinary and aromatic
plants and seeds

SPECIALTY BOTTLE
(206) 382-1100
www.specialtybottle.com
Online store; bottles and jars

STOKES SEEDS
(800) 396-9238
www.stokesseeds.com
Online store

GENERAL INFORMATION

BOTANIC GARDENS CONSERVATION INTERNATIONAL
www.bgci.org
A global network of botanic gardens working for
plant conservation and undertaking medicinal
plant research around the world

EVERGREEN NATIVE PLANT DATABASE
www.evergreen.ca
A volunteer-run searchable database that lists
plants by Canadian province, species or
particular attribute

HERB SOCIETY OF AMERICA
www.herbsociety.org
Plant profiles and herb growing advice

MONROVIA
www.monrovia.com
Garden designing instructions, information on
gardening and soil upkeep, garden center
finder

NATIONAL GARDENING ASSOCIATION
www.garden.org
Database of articles on plants and gardening;
plant finder and information

NATIONAL WILDLIFE FOUNDATION
www.nwf.org
Organization dedicated to conservation; offers
advice on how to grow an environmentally
friendly garden

NATURE CONSERVANCY CANADA
www.natureconservancy.ca
Information on how your garden can help
preserve the biodiversity and natural heritage
of Canada

UNITED STATES NATIONAL ARBORETUM
www.usna.usda.gov
Detailed information and news about
horticulture in the United States and hardiness
zone map of North America

INDEX

ACKNOWLEDGMENTS

AUTHOR'S ACKNOWLEDGMENTS

Working on this book and the UK TV series has been a huge adventure. Behind the scenes there has been a whole team of people whose untiring efforts have helped make it all possible. First, a huge thank you is in order to Lisa Edwards at the BBC for taking a chance on the idea. Equally, all the team at Silver River (you know who you are) have been absolutely terrific. I've never seen such passion and dedication, particularly when following me around wet fields in the cold rain! Liz at the University of Reading has been a true star with her pharmaceutical genius, and of course a huge thank you to my agent, Fiona, for her unending patience. I am also greatly indebted to HarperCollins for putting together this brilliant book. I had great fun working on it with them. Last, a major thanks to all my family and friends for believing in me—and putting up with my geeky plant obsession all these years.

PUBLISHERS' ACKNOWLEDGMENTS

The publishers would like to thank Timothy Dunn of Timothy Dunn Florists for a fabulous selection of flowers; Ginkgo Gardens for their help with photography; Peter Jarrett of Middlesex University for providing photographs from the university's Herbal Medicine Garden; and Kathryn Lwin Brooks of the Archway Clinic of Herbal Medicine.

PHOTOGRAPHY CREDITS

All photographs other than those listed below have been provided by Noel Murphy. Garden Picture Library 180R, 181L, 191L, 212L; iStock 157L, 159R, 174L, 185R, 187, 207L; Peter Jarrett (Medicinal Herb Garden of Middlesex University) 159L, 161R, 177R, 179R, 184L, 185L, 194R, 197L, 200L, 204L, 213R; Shutterstock 157R, 160L, 161L, 165R, 166L, 166R, 167L, 168R, 169R, 170, 171L, 173, 189L, 190L, 190R, 191R, 193R, 194L, 196R, 203R, 205R, 206R, 207R, 211L, 215L, 215R; William Shaw 162R, 168L.